125 Best
Gluten-Free
Recipes

Donna Washburn
and Heather Butt

Robert
ROSE

125 Best Gluten-Free Recipes
Text copyright © 2003 Donna Washburn and Heather Butt
Photographs copyright © 2003 Robert Rose Inc.

For complete cataloguing information, see page 184.

Disclaimer
The recipes in this book have been carefully tested. To the best of our knowledge, they are
safe and nutritious for ordinary use and users. All the recipes within this book are gluten-free
according to the Canadian Celiac Association dietary guidelines and based on reasonable
research for accuracy at the time of writing. For those people with food or other allergies,
or who have special food requirements or health issues, please read the suggested contents
of each recipe carefully and determine whether or not they may create a problem for you.
All recipes are used at the risk of the consumer.

   We cannot be responsible for any hazards, loss or damage that may occur as a result
of any recipe use.

   For those with special needs, allergies, requirements or health problems, in the event
of any doubt, please contact your medical adviser prior to the use of any recipe.

Design & Production: PageWave Graphics Inc.
Editor: Carol Sherman
Copy Editor: Deborah Aldcorn
Recipe Tester: Jennifer Mackenzie
Photography: Mark T. Shapiro
Food Stylist: Kate Bush
Props Stylist: Charlene Ericson
Color Scans: Colour Technologies

Cover image: Chocolate Fudge Cake (page 140) with Orange Frosting (page 156)

We acknowledge the financial support of the Government of Canada through the Book Publishing
Industry Development Program (BPIDP) for our publishing activities.

Published by: Robert Rose Inc.
120 Eglinton Ave. E., Suite 1000, Toronto, Ontario, Canada M4P 1E2
Tel: (416) 322-6552   Fax: (416) 322-6936

Printed in Canada
1 2 3 4 5 6 7 8 9 10   GP   09 08 07 06 05 04 03

We dedicate this book to those who live
with gluten intolerance and to their families.
We developed these recipes with you in mind.
We hope we help make dining a more
enjoyable experience.

Foreword

This cookbook was written for those who have been medically diagnosed with celiac disease or dermatitis herpetiformis and who must follow a strict gluten-free diet for life. Those with wheat or other grain allergies will also find this cookbook very useful.

Celiac disease, or gluten-sensitive enteropathy, is a genetic, autoimmune disease that leads to a permanent intolerance to gluten. Dermatitis herpetiformis is a related condition that primarily affects the skin and results in an intensely itchy, burning rash, but it can also damage the gastrointestinal tract, as can celiac disease. There is no cure for these diseases, nor is there a simple pill to pop. Treatment for both is a strict gluten-free diet for life.

When an individual with celiac disease ingests any amount of the protein gluten, it results in inflammatory damage to the villous lining of the small intestine, leading to the malabsorption of nutrients needed for good health. Left untreated, this can eventually result in severe malnutrition and an increased risk for other diseases, including lymphoma and osteoporosis. Individuals with celiac disease can also develop other associated conditions, including insulin dependent diabetes, thyroid disease, miscarriages and infertility, attention deficit disorder, and neural tube defects in newborns.

While a gluten-free diet may sound easy in principle, many individuals with celiac disease find it to be both difficult and frustrating because there are many hidden sources of gluten. Gluten is a storage protein found in the grains, wheat, rye, barley, and triticale and possibly oats or their derivatives. Grains that contain gluten are used widely in commercial products and include wheat starch, starch fillers, vegetable gums, hydrolyzed vegetable or plant proteins, seasonings, flavorings and malt flavoring, to name only a few. Grocery shopping is both challenging and time consuming. Those with celiac disease or dermatitis herpetiformis must be diligent at reading and interpreting product labels to search out the hidden sources of gluten. Many manufacturers now provide gluten-free products. While this is a real benefit for those following this diet, the downside is these products are often expensive; they may not taste exactly like their gluten-containing counterparts; and they are not enriched with vitamins and minerals.

The Canadian Celiac Association advises that if you think you may have celiac disease and are considering being tested, do not begin a gluten-free diet until all tests have been performed properly and the diagnosis is confirmed.

Many people who follow a gluten-free diet have chosen to go "back to the basics" by making their own baked goods. There are several excellent gluten-free alternatives that can be used to replace wheat. These include amaranth, arrowroot, buckwheat, corn bran, corn flour, corn meal, cornstarch, flax, legume flours (bean, garbanzo or chickpea, garfava, lentil and pea) millet, potato flour and potato starch, quinoa, rice bran, rice polishings, rice flours (white, brown, sweet), sago, sorghum, soy flour, sweet potato flour, tapioca and teff.

With this gluten-free cookbook and a little patience and practice, anyone can master the art of cooking gluten-free.

Mavis Molloy, RDN
Member of the professional advisory board for the Canadian Celiac Association

Celiac disease is a medical condition in which the lining of the small intestine is damaged by a substance called gluten. The tiny, hair-like projections that line the walls of the intestine, called villi, become flattened. As a result, there is less surface area available for the absorption of nutrients from foods. This can make the risk for malnutrition high.

Symptoms of celiac disease typically include weakness, weight loss, diarrhea and anemia. There can be variations in the symptoms and their severity, making the path to a firm diagnosis difficult. A true diagnosis can only be made after an intestinal biopsy has been performed. While it might be tempting to try to eliminate gluten in an effort to relieve some symptoms, the diet should not be started until after the biopsy. To follow the diet before a biopsy is performed may lead to a missed diagnosis and improper treatment recommendations.

A related condition, dermatitis herpetiformis, is a chronic skin condition that involves severe skin itch, burning and rash. Again, an intestinal biopsy is required to confirm the diagnosis since the changes to the lining of the small intestine are identical.

A gluten-free diet helps the small intestine to heal, allowing for normal nutrient digestion and absorption. It also helps relieve the symptoms of celiac disease and dermatitis herpetiformis.

Gluten is the storage protein of many grains, including wheat, oats, rye and barley. These foods, as well as anything made with them, must be eliminated and this requires a careful review of all labels. While removing gluten from the diet often results in a dramatic improvement in symptoms, the prospect of doing so can be overwhelming.

Initially, the challenge lies with determining what foods should be avoided. Consulting with a registered dietitian can help a celiac live with a gluten-free diet, while making sure that it is healthy, well-balanced and, most important, enjoyable.

One of the most difficult challenges is continuing to follow the diet after symptoms have disappeared. A person with celiac disease must be "gluten-free for life" because an intake of even small amounts of gluten can be damaging. Just a little gluten may not lead to the return of symptoms, but it will still cause intestinal damage. Wavering from the diet increases the risk of other health problems, including specific cancers of the small intestine.

Another challenge is getting other people to take the condition seriously. Food allergy and food intolerance are becoming commonplace words and they may not carry the same meaning for everyone. A food allergy triggers an immune response in the body and the results can be severe and even life threatening. On the other hand, a food intolerance occurs when someone cannot digest part of a certain food. Most people with a food intolerance can eat a small amount of the problem item without too much difficulty, making it less serious in most cases. However, while celiac disease and dermatitis herpetiformis are, in fact, an intolerance to gluten, intake of even a small amount can have a damaging effect. This is truly something be taken seriously.

When a family member has celiac disease, this has usually meant cooking a separate meal for him or her. Gluten-free foods do not have to be plain or boring. In fact, this cookbook offers many suggestions for healthy, tasty meals that the whole family can enjoy. They also just happen to be gluten-free. What could be better? It boosts the morale of the person with celiac disease to know that the whole family is enjoying the same meal and saves time for the cook — only one meal to prepare!

As a registered dietitian who has worked with clients with celiac disease, I wholeheartedly welcome these new gluten-free recipes. I am sure that those with the condition will also enjoy the recipes and new ideas of this book.

Leanna Knox-Kinsman B.Sc., RD
Nutrition Focus

Acknowledgments

This book has had the support and assistance of many from its inception to the final reality. We want to thank those who helped us along the way.

Our thanks to the following for supplying products for recipe development: Doug Yuen, Dainty Foods, for rice, white and brown rice flour and rice bran; George Birinyi Jr., Grain Process Enterprises Ltd., for arrowroot, potato and tapioca starches, xanthan gum, white and brown rice flour and yellow pea flour; Kingsmill Foods for Egg Replacer; Vicki van As and Hot-Kid for rice crackers; Diana Phillips and Notta Pasta for rice pasta; Jim Grey, Casco, for corn syrup and cornstarch; Connie Priest-Brown, Compass Food Sales, for arrowroot, tapioca and potato starches; Dennis Gilliam, Bobs Red Mill, for introducing us to sorghum flour (Jowar) and providing this and other gluten-free products; the employee-owners, The Baker's Catalogue of King Arthur Flour Company, for nut flours, xanthan gum, English muffin rings, hamburger and hotdog baking pans; Margaret Hudson, Burnbrae Farms Ltd., for Naturegg Simply Whites, Break Free and Omega Pro liquid eggs; Wendi Hiebert, Ontario Egg Producers, for whole shell eggs and Maryline Demandre, Lallamand Inc., for InstaFerm® (fermipan®) yeast.

Thank you to the many manufacturers of bread machines who continue to supply the latest models to our test kitchen; Philips Electronics Ltd, Proctor Silex/Hamilton Beach, GE, Toastmaster, Breadman, Black and Decker, Charlescraft and Zojirushi.

A huge thank you to the members of our focus group who faithfully and tirelessly tasted and tested gluten-free recipes and products from the beginning to end of recipe development. Your comments, suggestions and critical analysis were invaluable and helped make this a better book. Thanks to Susan Crapper, Rita Purcell, Carol Coulter, Debra Rice, Jim Morton, Larry Bomford, Barbara Wahn, Sue and Deanna Jennett. You'll be pleased to see we listened and incorporated your suggestions.

Information and assistance was invaluable from Linda, Elsie and Mike of New Horizons.

A special thank you to Leanna Knox-Kinsman, RD, and Mavis Molloy, RDN, for their contributions to the foreword. Mavis, thank you for reviewing our manuscript for accuracy in following the Canadian Celiac Association dietary guidelines.

We want to express our appreciation to photographer Mark Shapiro; food stylist Kate Bush and prop stylist Charlene Ericson. Thank you for making our gluten-free photographs so enticing. Once again, we enjoyed baking for the photo shoot.

Bob Dees, our publisher, and Marian Jarkovich, sales and marketing manager, at Robert Rose, deserve special thanks for their ongoing support.

To Andrew Smith, Daniella Zanchetta and Joseph Gisini of PageWave Graphics, thank you for working through this cookbook's design, layout and production.

To Carol Sherman, our editor, you're great! Your efficient, organized style and open communication made working with you a pleasure.

Thank you to our families, husbands, sons, daughters-in-law and grandsons. You helped bring balance to our lives when we became too focused on our work.

Donna J. Washburn and Heather L. Butt

Table of Contents

Introduction

As professional home economists, we both have university degrees in our field of study and have taught nutrition, food theory and food safety at community colleges. Almost 10 years ago, we formed Quality Professional Services to develop recipes for bread machine manufacturers and over time for yeast companies. Our cookbooks include *Canada's/America's Best Bread Machine Baking Recipes*, *More of Canada's/America's Best Bread Machine Baking Recipes* and *125 Best Quick Bread Recipes*. We also publish an international newsletter, *The Bread Basket*, for bread machine owners and we manage a toll-free consumer information line.

We have received numerous requests for gluten-free recipes for the bread machine, desserts and treats. Although no one in our families has a gluten intolerance, we have both dealt with allergies. Donna had to read labels for years while baking for a young son with a wheat allergy. She has first-hand knowledge through her son of the importance of fitting in at a birthday party or carrying cookies to school without finding a bag of crumbs at lunch. At present, Heather's husband is learning to manage allergies.

Our knowledge of how gluten-free flours act in recipes was limited. We explored existing cookbooks, web sites and baking textbooks. We read labels and haunted grocery and health food stores. We visited ethnic grocery stores and trade shows to discover what products were readily available in all areas of the United States and Canada. From Vancouver to Nova Scotia to Texas, we set up focus groups and asked questions. We met and e-mailed celiacs who shared personal stories and food experiences.

We baked and baked and baked. We tasted and tested and delivered them to families with a celiac for tasting and evaluating. Our most common question was "Could this or does this contain gluten?" Lists of gluten-free foods were garnered from web sites and food companies and celiac associations.

Our aim was to develop recipes the whole family could enjoy. Our greatest reward came by e-mail. We had delivered a cake to a local celiac and she wrote, "I did not get to taste the Gingered Pumpkin Snacking Cake — my non-celiac husband ate the whole thing and left me a note pronouncing it 'very good.'"

Our focus groups offered suggestions and requests — everyone wanted recipes for tender pastry, lemon loaf, butter tart squares, cheesecake, carrot cake, a good white cake for birthdays and, of course — chocolate cake, chocolate cake, chocolate cake. We have included these old favorites as well as special-occasion recipes of trifle, galette and fresh fruit cobbler. They wanted breads and desserts. We have included muffins and cookies, breads and pasta.

We hope you contact us and let us know your thoughts and share with us how you personalized these recipes for your family's enjoyment. Tell us your favorites. We would appreciate your comments.

Donna and Heather

Quality Professional Services
1655 County Road 2
Mallorytown, Ontario K0E 1R0

or

P. O. Box 1382
Ogdensburg, New York 13669
phone/fax: 613-923-2116
email: *bread@ripnet.com*
website: *www.bestbreadrecipes.com*

The Gluten-Free Bake Shop

Baking is a science as well as an art. It is important to select the correct ingredients. Let's take a quick look at some of the ingredients available.

When both gluten-free and gluten-containing products are available, we've indicated by using a **GF** (gluten-free) beside the ingredient that this must be used.

FLOURS AND STARCHES

Baking with flours that do not contain gluten creates special problems for the baker, as it is the gluten that provides the cell structure in hearty yeast breads and light airy cakes. Over the last few years, the range of flours and starches readily available has expanded, as has the knowledge of working with them. It is necessary to combine flours and starches to balance flavor, texture, mouth feel and keeping quality in baked goods. Although you may find a specific combination of flours and starches repeated in several recipes, we have not selected one or two combinations to use in every recipe, but developed each on its own to give us the taste and baking qualities we desired.

The major flours and starches are described here. Information about others used in the book is explained in the Ingredient Glossary (see page 173). Unless otherwise specified, store all flours and starches in airtight containers away from heat and light. For more prolonged storage, freeze. Sift or mix flours and starches well before using.

Arrowroot Starch is the flavorless, fine, white powder of a West Indian plant. We use it in berry sauces as it thickens below the boiling point, giving a warm, clear shine. It must be mixed with a cold liquid before adding to hot liquids.

Bean Flour has more protein than other gluten-free flours, thus bread rises higher and the products are often more tender. It is usually combined with other flours because of its stronger flavor. We particularly like a sorghum/bean combination for recipes containing chocolate, molasses or applesauce. Bean flours absorb more moisture than other flours so you may need to adjust the liquid slightly when making substitutions.

It can be manufactured from a variety of beans, yielding both light and dark flours. Each results in its own flavor and texture. Use the dark with chocolate, pumpernickel, mock rye and the light for fruit breads and cakes or in place of soy flour. Many companies treat beans before grinding into flour to reduce the flatulent effects. The flour is then labeled micronized, processed, precooked or toasted.

Several varieties include garbanzo bean (chickpea), garbanzo-fava (garfava), which combines garbanzo beans and fava beans (a broad bean which tastes very sweet and buttery) and whole bean flour from Romano (cranberry) beans. Our recipes were developed with whole bean flour. All bean and pea flours are interchangeable in recipes.

Cornstarch is a flavorless, white powder, which thickens sauces to a clear, shiny finish. It begins to thicken at the boiling point then thins again if over-cooked. As it lumps easily, cornstarch must be mixed with a dry ingredient or made into a paste with a cold liquid before it is added slowly to a hot liquid. We use it in recipes where a glaze is required. It becomes quite thick when cold. If too much is used in a baked product, it leaves a starchy aftertaste.

Pea Flour is colorful and high in fiber. It is available as green pea flour and yellow pea flour. It can be substituted in recipes calling for whole bean flour.

Potato Starch (Potato Starch Flour) differs from Potato Flour. Potato flour is too heavy to use in significant amounts for gluten-free baking. When added in small amounts, potato starch adds lightness and moistness to baked goods. We like to double sift potato starch as it lumps more easily than other starches.

Rice Flour is not used alone in recipes but as the major flour combined with smaller amounts of starches such as potato or tapioca. Its bland flavor lets the delicate flavors of mild herbs and spices through. When either white or brown rice flour can be used, we just call for rice flour in the ingredient list. Several types available include the following:

Brown Rice Flour is not brown as the name implies, but a light creamy color that gives warmth to a Nutmeg Loaf or Banana Nut Muffins. It has a grainy texture and provides more fiber than white rice flour but is interchangeable in recipes. Because of the bran present, it must be refrigerated.

White Rice Flour is chosen when a traditional white color is expected such as White Cake, Sticky Bun Snacking Cake and Lemon Yogurt Scones.

Rice Bran adds fiber to the product. We use it in a Mock Date Bran Muffin. Store in the refrigerator because it may become rancid.

Sweet Rice Flour (Glutinous or Sticky Rice Flour) is made from high-starch, sticky, short-grain rice. Both brown and white rice varieties have a slightly sweet flavor and a sticky texture. It contains more starch than either brown or white rice flours so is not used as flour but as a thickener or in small amounts replacing regular rice flour to lighten products. There are two grades: one is beige, grainy, sandy-colored. The other is white, starchy, less expensive and is sticky and gooey. The less expensive works better. A small amount on the fingers or sprinkled on a board makes handling gluten-free dough such as Pizza Dough a lot easier.

Sorghum, known to some as Jowar, is a millet-like grain high in fiber, starch and protein and rich in fat-soluble and B-vitamins. Not as finely ground as other flours, it is gray-white with tan undertones. The higher sugar content gives a sweet product, which browns well when baked. The slightly nutty, savory, very earthy flavor may be too strong when a neutral-flavored flour is required. We enjoy baking it with pumpkin, molasses and rhubarb.

Soy Flour, high in protein, is yellow-beige in color with a nutty flavor. It is made from soybeans. Strong in flavor and aroma, it is used in combination with other flours and flavors such as peanut butter, banana and strong spices. You will notice the strong aroma when mixing the batter. This is not present in the baked product. The higher fat browns more quickly than the lower fat. Store the higher fat flour in the refrigerator.

Tapioca Starch (Tapioca Flour) is a slightly sweet, white, powdery-fine flour made from the cassava root. You often find it used in small amounts with rice flour as it helps sweeten. Sauce recipes require twice as much tapioca starch to thicken as with other starches but it thickens more as it cools. It is often used in coatings as it browns quickly.

LEAVENERS

Leaveners in cakes, quick breads and yeast breads produce carbon dioxide, which when heated, expands the cell-wall structure, resulting in a light, even texture. Baking powder, baking soda, yeast and beaten egg whites are the ones we used in this book.

Baking Powder is used in cakes, biscuits and muffins. However, it can become a problem as some baking powders contain wheat starch, which will be specified on the label. Gluten-free baking powder is available in some areas and can be substituted in equal amounts in recipes. If not available, here is a recipe you could use to make your own: In a small bowl, sift together 2 tsp (10 mL) cream of tartar, 2 tsp (10 mL) cornstarch or arrowroot starch and 1 tsp (5 mL) baking soda. Make only small amounts at a time and store in an airtight container.

Baking Soda is selected when an acid ingredient such as buttermilk, lemon juice or molasses is used. It keeps in the cupboard for up to 6 months.

Yeast is a tiny, single-celled organism that, given moisture, food and warmth, creates gas that is trapped in bread dough, causing it to rise. Bread Machine Yeast (Instant Yeast) is added directly to the dry ingredients of breads. We use this yeast rather than Active Dry, as it does not need to be activated in water before using. Store in the freezer in an airtight container for up to 2 years.

Beaten Egg Whites Gluten-free cakes can be made even lighter in texture by separating the eggs in the recipe, adding the yolks with the other liquids or creaming with the fat and sugar. The beaten whites are folded in after the dry ingredients and liquids are combined with the creamed mixture.

HANDLING GLUTEN-FREE FLOURS AND STARCHES

• Purchase flours and starches from reliable sources for consistent quality and to ensure that there is no risk from cross-contamination. Once you succeed with a particular product, either brand or quality, stick with it.

• Store flours and starches in plastic containers rather than the bags they are purchased in. Select square, stackable, airtight containers, with wide tops and tightly fitting lids to allow for ease of measuring of these powdery ingredients.

• Label all containers with easy-to-read permanent markers. It is impossible to tell the difference between some of the white starches by feel or appearance.

• Sift all flours and starches as you fill the containers rather than spending the time each time you bake. Stir with a spoon or a fork, just before measuring.

• Organize a baking corner where you keep a variety of dry ingredients (store only those necessary in the refrigerator). This could be a deep drawer or an overhead cupboard. Keep a set of dry ingredient measures and spoons, a metal spatula, a large metal spoon, a heat resistant spatula, a set of your most commonly used baking pans and a cooling rack within easy reach.

• Occasionally, you might require a pan previously used for baking a wheat flour recipe. Wash it carefully, as small particles can get trapped in corners. Watch pans with ridges such as the rim of a springform pan.

• Wear a mask if handling gluten-containing flours. They can become airborne and inhalation can lead to problems.

SUCCESSFUL GLUTEN-FREE BAKING

• Read the recipe before you begin and make sure you have all the ingredients you need.

• Preheat the oven to ensure even airflow around the baked goods. Place two pans, side by side, in the middle of the oven with at least 1-inch (2.5 cm) between the pans.

• Prepare the pan according to the recipe directions. Grease the pans with a vegetable spray, vegetable oil or shortening; never butter. Do this before you measure or mix.

• Prepare all ingredients before mixing. This includes zesting lemons, washing and snipping fresh herbs and grating cheese.

Follow the recipe for sizes or shapes of individual pieces for vegetables or fruit as cooking times are based on these.

• Use the "spoon lightly into the correct dry measure, heap the top and level once" method of measuring for accuracy and perfect products. Mix together all the flours, starches, leaveners and seasonings in a bowl or plastic bag. If lumpy, take the time to sift several times. Always sift dry ingredients if cocoa or confectioner's (icing) sugar is included. We like to use the plastic bag as it is easy to shake to mix the dry ingredients.

• Follow all times exactly. Set an extra kitchen timer as 4 minutes seems forever as you are beating bread dough.

• Select the correct pan size for the recipe. If the pan is too large, the baked good may burn within the recipe baking time.

• Let the batter or dough stand at room temperature for 30 minutes before baking. The final product will be lighter in texture and more tender.

• Check the mixer manual for recommended settings when mixing, creaming or beating; the speed is important for the quality of the finished product.

• To see whether your dish is done, check at the shorter recommended, baking time of the recipe. The time may vary depending on your oven and the material and finish of the baking pan used.

• Unless otherwise recommended do not double recipes. It is better to make up several bags of dry ingredients and label the contents for baking later. Gluten-free products are often at their best when freshly prepared.

• Purchase a bread machine to be used only for gluten-free baking to avoid the risk of cross-contamination.

CHOOSING YOUR BAKING PANS

We recommend using shiny metal pans made from aluminum or tin. These reflect heat away from the baked product so that it browns evenly, but not too quickly. Insulated pans require extra baking time to brown, while foods baked in dark-colored pans brown more quickly, requiring less baking time.

Glass baking dishes conduct and retain heat, resulting in thicker, darker crusts. If you use this type, reduce the baking temperature by about 25°F (20°C). For example, if the recipe says to bake at 350°F (180°C), reduce the oven temperature to 325°F (160°C).

Similarly, we have found that metal baking pans with a nonstick finish also require a lower baking temperature. When recipes were baked at the standard 350°F (180°C), the crusts were darker and thicker. The loaves browned too quickly and were frequently burnt by the time the centers were baked. So be sure you know what type of pan you have and adjust your oven temperature accordingly.

For best results, it is important to use the size of pan specifically called for in the recipe. We tested and baked all our quick bread recipes in 9-by 5-inch (2 L) loaf pans. Most baked in 8-by 4-inch (1.5 L) pans, as well. Just be sure you only fill the pan about three-quarters full. This allows baked goods to bake evenly and prevents batter from overflowing the pan. As a rule, thicker batters rise less than thinner batters. So, the thicker the batter, the fuller the pan can be.

Tasty Beginnings

Recipes to whet your appetite or to serve as a meal on their own.

❧ Just for Kids ❧

- It is important that young people who suffer from celiac disease feel part of the group and not different. All decisions should be made keeping this in mind, while ensuring the diet is strictly followed.

- Teach! Teach! Teach! Don't make decisions for even the youngest child. Every time a new food is selected or served, casually explain why it can or cannot be tolerated. Stress the positive. Soon the questions will come from the child. It is important for children with celiac disease to know that the parent will not always be with them. "When I was too young to read," says 11-year-old Deanna Jennett, "I wore a MedicAlert bracelet. Whenever adults offered me food, I could ask them if I should have it because of what my bracelet said." Teach them that "if in doubt, do without."

- When a school-aged child is invited to sleep over or to attend a birthday party, call ahead to ask about the menu and to explain to the parents the child's dietary restrictions. It's important to send something similar. You may also want to send along gluten-free treats such as Chocolate Chip Cookies (see recipe, page 160) that all children can enjoy. When sending individual pizzas or individual foods, wrap them in foil so they can be reheated without cross-contamination.

- Speak to your child's class and explain why your child cannot eat what the others do and why they cannot share. Take along a few gluten-free treats to share with the class. You will find others in the class with special dietary needs and soon the youngsters' natural curiosity will speed along the discussion. We really liked the way Deanna educated her peers about her intolerance to gluten. "I made a model of the surface of the intestine for a science project. I used clay and stuck small pieces of wool in it like hair. I demonstrated in front of my class how the 'hairs' were destroyed by gluten and since the 'hairs' absorbed the nutrition from the food, they realized how serious it was for me to not have any gluten."

- Grocery shop with the young celiac child. Show the importance of reading every label every time. It takes longer, but is certainly worth the effort and even a young pre-teen can recognize ingredients to avoid. "One of the ways I learned to read was by reading labels," states Deanna, diagnosed when she was five years old. "Sometimes, Mum would take something off the shelf and ask me if it was safe. It was a bit of a game."

- When it is a communal dish, such as salsa and chips or vegetables and dip, make sure celiac children take their food first. They know they can't share food with others.

Broccoli-Cheddar Cornbread

**MAKES 9
SQUARE PIECES**

This tasty cornbread is ideal for entertaining. Cut into bite-size pieces, it can be served hot or cold as an hors d'oeuvre. It's also great for family meals.

TIP
Bake in a 2-quart (2 L) ovenproof casserole dish. Reduce baking temperature to 325°F (160°C). Serve hot, directly from the oven.

VARIATION
Substitute chopped red bell pepper for half the onions.

Preheat oven to 350°F (180°C)
9-inch (2.5 L) square baking pan, lightly greased

1 cup	cornmeal	250 mL
1 cup	rice flour	250 mL
¼ cup	potato starch	50 mL
¼ cup	tapioca starch	50 mL
1½ tsp	xanthan gum	7 mL
1 tbsp	GF baking powder	15 mL
1 tsp	baking soda	5 mL
½ tsp	salt	2 mL
1 cup	chopped onions	250 mL
¾ cup	shredded old Cheddar cheese	175 mL
¼ cup	freshly grated Parmesan cheese	50 mL
1 cup	broccoli florets	250 mL
1 tsp	cider vinegar	5 mL
3	eggs	3
2 tbsp	honey	25 mL
1	can (14 oz/398 mL) cream-style corn	1

1. In a large bowl, stir together cornmeal, rice flour, potato starch, tapioca starch, xanthan gum, baking powder, baking soda and salt. Stir in onions, Cheddar, Parmesan and broccoli. Set aside.

2. In a separate bowl, using an electric mixer, beat vinegar, eggs and honey until combined. Stir in corn.

3. Pour corn mixture over dry ingredients and stir just until combined. Spoon into prepared pan. Allow to stand for 30 minutes.

4. Bake in preheated oven for 35 to 45 minutes or until a cake tester inserted in the center comes out clean. Serve hot.

Lavosh

Keep this thin, low-fat, crisp Armenian flatbread on hand to serve as a snack with fresh vegetables, for dipping in salsa or with soups and salads.

TIPS

The thinner the dough is spread, the more authentic the cracker will be.

Store crackers in an airtight container for up to 2 months. If necessary, crisp the Lavosh in the oven, before serving.

Large baking sheet, lightly greased

¾ cup	brown rice flour	175 mL
⅓ cup	tapioca starch	75 mL
1 tsp	granulated sugar	5 mL
1½ tsp	xanthan gum	7 mL
1½ tsp	bread machine or instant yeast	7 mL
½ tsp	salt	2 mL
¾ cup	water	175 mL
1 tsp	cider vinegar	5 mL
1 tbsp	vegetable oil	15 mL
¼ cup	sesame seeds	50 mL
1 to 2 tbsp	sweet rice flour	15 to 25 mL

BREAD MACHINE METHOD

1. In a large bowl or plastic bag, combine brown rice flour, tapioca starch, sugar, xanthan gum, yeast and salt. Mix well and set aside.

2. Pour water, vinegar and oil into the bread machine baking pan. Select the Dough Cycle. Allow the liquids to mix until combined.

3. Gradually, add the dry ingredients as the bread machine is mixing, scraping with a rubber spatula while adding. Try to incorporate all the dry ingredients within 1 to 2 minutes. Allow the bread machine to complete the cycle.

MIXER METHOD

1. In a large bowl or plastic bag, combine brown rice flour, tapioca starch, sugar, xanthan gum, yeast and salt. Mix well and set aside.

2. Pour water, vinegar and oil into the large bowl of a heavy-duty mixer.

3. Using paddle attachment with the mixer on the lowest speed, slowly add the dry ingredients until combined. With a rubber spatula, scrape the bottom and sides of the bowl. With the mixer on medium speed, beat for 4 minutes.

FOR BOTH METHODS

4. Sprinkle prepared baking sheet with half the sesame seeds. Remove dough to prepared sheet. Sprinkle generously with 1 tbsp (15 mL) sweet rice flour. Place waxed paper, generously dusted with sweet rice flour, on top of the dough. Gently pat the waxed paper to spread the dough, lifting and re-dusting frequently to check the dough thickness. Carefully remove the waxed paper. Sprinkle with remaining sesame seeds. Press lightly into dough. Bake in 375°F (190°C) preheated oven for 20 to 25 minutes or until lightly browned. Remove from oven. Allow to cool, then break into large pieces.

Crispy Cheese Crackers

MAKES 10 DOZEN CRACKERS

Try to eat just one of these delicious morsels! If you make a double batch, you'll be able to hide some in the freezer. Use them as a base for hors d'oeuvres as a well as a cracker to serve with a soup or salad.

TIPS

To prevent crackers from softening, store in an airtight container for up to 2 months.

❧

You can also freeze the logs for 1 month. Thaw in refrigerator before slicing.

VARIATION

Purchase a shredded Tex-Mex mix of Mozzarella, Cheddar and Monterey Jack with jalapeños and substitute it for the Cheddar. Check for gluten before you purchase a packaged shredded cheese mix.

Baking sheet, greased or lined with parchment

1 cup	brown rice flour	250 mL
¾ cup	sorghum flour	175 mL
¼ cup	cornstarch	50 mL
1 tsp	xanthan gum	5 mL
Pinch	cayenne pepper	Pinch
½ tsp	paprika	2 mL
½ cup	shredded old Cheddar cheese	125 mL
½ cup	freshly grated Parmesan cheese	125 mL
⅓ cup	butter, softened	75 mL
⅔ cup	GF sour cream	150 mL

1. In a large bowl, combine brown rice flour, sorghum flour, cornstarch, xanthan gum, cayenne pepper, paprika, Cheddar and Parmesan. Mix well and set aside.

2. In another bowl, using an electric mixer, cream butter and sour cream. Gradually beat in dry ingredients, mixing until blended. Squeeze handfuls of mixture to form into 6 logs, each 1½ inches (4 cm) in diameter. Wrap in plastic wrap and refrigerate overnight. Allow to stand at room temperature for 15 to 20 minutes.

3. Cut logs into ⅛-inch (3 mm) thick slices. Place on prepared baking sheet. Place at least 1 inch (2.5 cm) apart on baking sheet. Bake in 375°F (190°C) preheated oven for 6 to 8 minutes or until golden brown. One extra minute of baking can burn these thin crackers. Remove immediately. Serve warm or transfer onto racks to cool completely.

Holiday Cheese Balls

The red, green and orange flecks of the bell peppers make this an ideal appetizer to serve at a holiday open house.

TIP

If the mixture is too soft to form into balls, refrigerate for 10 minutes before shaping. Use the cheese balls right away or freeze for up to 4 weeks to serve at a later time. They keep in the refrigerator for up to 1 week.

VARIATIONS

Make one large ball, if preferred.

～

Roll in snipped fresh parsley or decorate with whole unblanched almonds, instead of the pecans.

8 oz	cream cheese, softened	250 g
4 oz	blue cheese, crumbled	125 g
2 tsp	prepared horseradish	10 mL
3 to 4	drops hot pepper sauce	3 to 4
1	clove garlic, minced	1
3	green onions, finely chopped	3
1/2 cup	chopped red, orange and/or yellow bell pepper	125 mL
2 cups	shredded old Cheddar cheese	500 mL
2 to 3 cups	finely chopped pecans	500 to 750 mL

1. In a large bowl, combine cream cheese, blue cheese, horseradish, hot pepper sauce to taste and garlic. Set aside.

2. In a microwave-safe bowl, combine green onions and bell peppers. Microwave, covered, on High for 1 minute. (Or steam in a covered saucepan over low heat for 2 to 3 minutes or until tender-crisp.)

3. Combine onion-pepper mixture with Cheddar cheese. Fold into cream cheese mixture. Divide in half and form into 2 balls. Wrap in plastic wrap and chill for 30 minutes. Roll in pecans. Serve on a platter with crackers.

Broccoli-Cheddar Soup

SERVES 4 TO 6

The tiny crisp broccoli florets add a slight crunch to this creamy soup. It's perfect to serve on a cold winter day.

TIPS

Select broccoli with thin, slender stalks. Two medium bunches yield 6 cups (1.5 L) chopped. Peel the stalks, if they are woody.

∾

For a chunky soup, do not purée.

∾

Use either a homemade gluten-free chicken stock or a commercial gluten-free chicken stock powder.

∾

You can use a gluten-free vegetable stock for a vegetarian version.

VARIATIONS

Substitute cauliflower for all or part of the broccoli.

∾

Try thyme, marjoram or tarragon instead of the basil.

2 tsp	vegetable oil	10 mL
1½ cups	chopped leeks, white and light green parts only	375 mL
1 cup	diced potato	250 mL
2	cloves garlic, minced	2
4 cups	diced broccoli stalks and florets (see Tips, left)	1 L
4 cups	GF chicken stock	1 L
1 tbsp	chopped fresh basil	15 mL
2 cups	chopped broccoli florets	500 mL
	Salt and freshly ground black pepper	
1 cup	shredded old Cheddar cheese	250 mL

1. In a large saucepan, heat oil over medium heat. Add leeks, potato and garlic. Cook, stirring frequently, until leeks are tender. Add diced broccoli and stock. Simmer, covered, for 15 minutes or until vegetables are tender.

2. In a food processor or blender, purée in batches. Return to saucepan. Add basil and chopped broccoli florets. Simmer until broccoli is tender. Season with salt and pepper to taste. Stir in cheese just before serving.

Mushroom Wild Rice Chowder

SERVES 4

Select shiitake, oyster or button mushrooms to give this thick soup a new twist each time.

TIPS

About 2 stalks of celery make ½ cup (125 mL) when chopped.

∾

The half-and-half cream separates and curdles if the soup is allowed to boil.

VARIATIONS

Use gluten-free vegetable stock for the gluten-free chicken stock.

∾

Substitute milk for the half-and-half cream.

1 cup	wild rice, uncooked	250 mL
2 tbsp	butter	25 mL
4 cups	sliced fresh mushrooms	1 L
½ cup	chopped celery (see Tips, left)	125 mL
1 cup	chopped leeks, white and light green parts only	250 mL
3	shallots, finely chopped	3
2	cloves garlic, minced	2
4 cups	GF chicken stock	1 L
1 tsp	dried marjoram	5 mL
¼ tsp	freshly ground black pepper	1 mL
1 cup	half-and-half (10%) cream	250 mL

1. Rinse wild rice under cold, running water. Drain and set aside.
2. In a large saucepan, melt butter over medium heat. Add mushrooms, celery, leeks, shallots and garlic. Cook, stirring frequently, until vegetables are tender. Add stock, rice, marjoram and pepper. Simmer, covered, for 45 to 60 minutes or until rice is tender. Slowly stir in cream. Heat through but do not boil.

Sweet Potato Soup

SERVES 4

This thick soup evokes the vibrant colors of autumn. Serve it along with the Ciabatta (see recipe, page 38).

TIP

If you prefer a thinner soup, add extra vegetable stock just before serving.

VARIATIONS

Use basil or nutmeg instead of ginger. Add a small amount at a time, simmer for a couple of minutes and taste.

∾

Substitute winter squash or carrots for all or part of the sweet potato.

∾

Add 2 large peeled and diced apples with the sweet potatoes.

2 tsp	vegetable oil	10 mL
1 1/2 cups	chopped onions, about 2 medium	375 mL
1 cup	diced potato	250 mL
2	cloves garlic, minced	2
4 cups	diced sweet potato, about 1 1/4 lbs (625 g)	1 L
4 cups	GF vegetable stock	1 L
1 1/2 tsp	ground ginger	7 mL
	Salt and freshly ground black pepper	

1. In a large saucepan, heat oil over medium heat. Add onions, potato and garlic. Cook, stirring frequently, until onions are tender.

2. Add sweet potato and vegetable stock. Simmer, covered, for 20 minutes or until vegetables are tender. Add ginger.

3. In a food processor or blender, purée soup in batches. Heat to just below boiling. Season to taste with salt and pepper.

Greek Pasta Salad

SERVES 4 TO 6

Enjoy this colorful salad mid-summer with garden-fresh cucumbers and tomatoes.

TIPS

An 8-oz (227 g) package contains 4 cups (1 L) gluten-free pasta.

～

We tried several types of gluten-free pastas and preferred a rice fusilli with rice bran. Experiment to find what you like the best.

VARIATION

Substitute small zucchini for the cucumber — no need to peel.

DRESSING

½ cup	extra virgin olive oil	125 mL
3 tbsp	freshly squeezed lemon juice	45 mL
¼ cup	fresh oregano leaves, snipped	50 mL
4	cloves garlic, minced	4
¼ tsp	salt	1 mL
Pinch	freshly ground black pepper	Pinch

SALAD

1 cup	GF pasta, macaroni, rotini or fusilli (see Tips, left)	250 mL
4	plum tomatoes, cut in wedges	4
1	seedless cucumber, cut in half lengthwise, then sliced	1
1	yellow or orange bell pepper, cut into ¼-inch (0.5 cm) strips	1
½	small red onion, cut in rings	½
½ cup	sliced Kalamata olives	125 mL
4 oz	feta cheese, broken into chunks	125 g

1. *Dressing:* In a small bowl, whisk together olive oil, lemon juice, oregano, garlic, salt and pepper until mixed.

2. *Salad:* In a large saucepan, cook pasta in boiling water according to package instructions or until just firm to the bite. Rinse in cold water and drain. Place in a large bowl.

3. Add tomatoes, cucumber, bell pepper, onion and olives. Pour dressing over pasta and vegetables. Toss lightly to coat. Chill several hours or overnight. Place in serving bowl then add feta and toss.

Grilled Chicken Mandarin Salad with Sweet-and-Sour Dressing

SERVES 4

This traditional salad has become popular at quick-service restaurants. Enjoy it at home. Try the variations for a different salad every time.

TIP

The small delicate spinach leaves are milder than the mature ones. Also referred to as young spinach.

VARIATIONS

Double the dressing recipe and use half to marinate the raw chicken for at least 30 minutes in the refrigerator before grilling. Be sure to drain the chicken and discard the marinade.

∽

To make this a warm salad, heat the dressing to just below boiling before pouring it over that salad topped with freshly grilled chicken. Perfect during cool weather.

SWEET-AND-SOUR DRESSING

¼ cup	vegetable oil	50 mL
2 tbsp	granulated sugar	25 mL
2 tbsp	white vinegar	25 mL
2 tbsp	snipped fresh parsley	25 mL
¼ tsp	salt	1 mL
Pinch	freshly ground black pepper	Pinch
2 to 3 drops	hot pepper sauce	2 to 3 drops

SALAD

6 oz	baby spinach (see Tip, left)	175 g
1 cup	sliced celery	250 mL
¼ cup	thinly sliced green onions	50 mL
1	can (10 oz/284 mL) mandarin orange segments, drained	1
4	chicken breasts, grilled, cut into ¼-inch (0.5 cm) strips	4
	Caramelized Almonds (see recipe, page 25)	

1. *Sweet-and-Sour Dressing:* In a small bowl, whisk together oil, sugar, vinegar, parsley, salt, pepper and hot pepper sauce. Set aside for at least 1 hour. Refrigerate for up to 3 weeks.

2. *Salad:* In a salad bowl, toss together spinach, celery, green onions and mandarin orange segments.

3. Pour dressing over the salad and toss lightly. Top with grilled chicken strips and sprinkle with Caramelized Almonds.

Caramelized Almonds

MAKES ½ CUP (125 ML)

½ cup	slivered almonds	125 mL
2 tbsp	granulated sugar	25 mL

For those who like an added crunch on their salad, make these nuts ahead of time to sprinkle on Grilled Chicken Mandarin Salad (see recipe, page 24) or another one of your favorite salads.

1. In a small frying pan, cook almonds and sugar over medium heat, stirring constantly, until sugar is melted and almonds are coated and lightly browned. Set aside to cool then separate. Store in an airtight container for up to 3 months.

TIPS

Remember, melted sugar is hotter than deep fat. Remove the pan from the heat just as the sugar melts and begins to darken, as it burns very easily.

❧

Double the recipe so there is lots to nibble on while enjoying a glass of wine or to serve with Beef and Pepper Stir-Fry (see recipe, page 31).

VARIATION

Substitute pecan halves, pine nuts or a mixture of nuts for the almonds.

Shrimp Caesar Salad with Garlic Croutons

SERVES 4

Restaurant sales of Caesar salads increase daily. Carry your own Dijon dressing and gluten-free croutons or make them to serve at home.

TIPS

Extra salad dressing can be stored in the refrigerator for up to 3 weeks.

❧

For a milder mustard flavor, reduce the Dijon mustard to 1 tbsp (15 mL).

DIJON DRESSING

¾ cup	extra virgin olive oil	175 mL
⅓ cup	freshly squeezed lemon juice	75 mL
2 to 3 tbsp	Dijon mustard	25 to 45 mL

SALAD

1	head romaine lettuce, torn into bite-size pieces	1
8 oz	large shrimp, cooked, peeled and deveined	250 g
	Garlic Croutons (see recipe, below)	

1. *Dijon Dressing:* In a small bowl, whisk together olive oil, lemon juice and Dijon mustard to taste. Set aside for at least 1 hour before serving to allow flavors to develop and blend.
2. *Salad:* In a large bowl, combine lettuce, shrimp and just enough dressing to moisten. Top with gluten-free garlic croutons.

Garlic Croutons

MAKES 5 DOZEN

This is a good way to use up gluten-free bread that you found in the freezer!

VARIATION

Either add dried herbs or make croutons from any of the bread recipes on pages 81 to 110.

Preheat oven to 375°F (190°C)

4	slices day-old GF bread, cut into 1-inch (2.5 cm) cubes	4
1 tbsp	extra virgin olive oil	15 mL
2	cloves garlic, minced	2

1. In a bowl, toss bread cubes with oil and garlic. Spread in a single layer on a baking sheet. Bake in preheated oven for 10 to 15 minutes or until crisp and golden, turning frequently. Cool completely then store in an airtight container.

Roasted Garlic with Sun-Dried Tomato Dressing

**MAKES 1½ CUPS
(375 ML)**

1	head garlic	1
1 cup	plain yogurt	250 mL
½ cup	GF sour cream	125 mL
½ cup	snipped sun-dried tomatoes	125 mL
¼ cup	snipped fresh parsley	50 mL

The colors of this dressing are reminiscent of the Mediterranean. Besides using it to dress a fresh green salad, enjoy it spread on a roast beef sandwich.

VARIATIONS

Substitute gluten-free mayonnaise for the gluten-free sour cream to turn this dressing into a dip.

∽

For a dill-flavored dressing, substitute ¼ cup (50 mL) snipped fresh dill for fresh parsley.

1. *To roast garlic:* Cut off top of head to expose clove tips. Drizzle with ¼ tsp (1 mL) olive oil and microwave on High for 70 seconds or until fork-tender. Or bake in a pie plate or baking dish at 375°F (190°C) for 15 to 20 minutes.

2. In a small bowl, stir together yogurt, sour cream, garlic, sun-dried tomatoes and parsley. Cover and refrigerate for a minimum of 2 hours to allow flavors to develop and blend. Refrigerate for up to 2 weeks. The longer the dip is refrigerated, the stronger the flavor and the deeper the color becomes.

Green Goddess Salad Dressing

MAKES 1 CUP (250 ML)

Attractive, colorful, contrasting flecks of green — this is the dressing everyone requests. Use as a dip on a tray with your favorite crudités. Serve as a dressing over potato, pasta or carrot coleslaw salads.

TIPS

This recipe can be halved or doubled, depending on the amount you require.

❧

For the best color, be sure to purchase fresh parsley.

1	small clove garlic	1
1	green onion	1
¼ cup	fresh parsley	50 mL
1½ tsp	dried tarragon or 1 to 2 tbsp (15 to 25 mL) snipped fresh	7 mL
½ cup	GF sour cream	125 mL
½ cup	plain yogurt	125 mL
1 tbsp	freshly squeezed lemon juice	15 mL

1. In a food processor, combine garlic, green onion, parsley, tarragon, sour cream, yogurt and lemon juice. Process until smooth. Cover and refrigerate for a minimum of 2 hours to allow flavors to develop and blend. Refrigerate for up to 2 weeks.

The Main Event

For casual weekend get-togethers, hurry-up weeknight suppers or special dinners, plan your menu around these beef, pork, poultry or seafood recipes. When dining in isn't on the menu, we've even offered a special guide to eating out.

∾ Eating Out ∾
Restaurants, Weddings and Banquets

• When planning to dine out, call the restaurant ahead, if possible, to find out whether it offers gluten-free entrées. If the staff seem hesitant with their answers, choose a different restaurant.

• Choose restaurants that specialize in seafood, Mexican, Indian and Thai foods. These may be cooked to order — broiling, stir-frying or steaming individual portions.

• Establish a rapport with two or three local restaurants. It is great to know that your foods will be prepared safely, without you having to talk with the server and kitchen staff every time you want to eat out.

• Speak with the chef or person in charge of the food preparation. Most people pay attention to and understand the word "allergic" rather than "intolerance." Explain the consequences of eating just a small amount of gluten. A good example could be that even eating from a plate from which a bun that contained gluten was removed, may cause a reaction that lasts for weeks.

• Ask the server to check whether or not the fries are cooked in the same oil as the chicken fingers or other batter-fried foods.

• Carry a restaurant allergy identification card to present to the server and kitchen staff. You can make your own and laminate it. Make several, as they are easy to misplace or leave behind.

• Wear a MedicAlert bracelet at all times. It is often easier to point to the bracelet when asking for special consideration in a restaurant than to explain why you have brought some of your own food with you.

• For a special occasion celebration, call ahead to inquire about the menu and its suitability for your diet. Make suggestions of ways that they can accommodate you easily. It may mean something as simple as serving you the greens undressed and you bringing your own gluten-free salad dressing. Fresh fruit is always a good dessert.

Beef and Pepper Stir-Fry

SERVES 4 TO 6

Is your family asking for Chinese food tonight? Serve this quick stir-fry over rice or gluten-free noodles.

TIPS

One 10-oz (284 mL) can of gluten-free stock can be substituted for 1¼ cups (300 mL) reconstituted gluten-free broth powder.

∾

For more tender beef, slice in thin strips across the grain. Slice while the beef is partially frozen. It's easier!

VARIATION

Steam 2 cups (500 mL) small broccoli florets to add with tomatoes. Substitute chicken or pork for the beef and gluten-free chicken stock or gluten-free vegetable stock for the gluten-free beef stock.

1¼ lbs	boneless sirloin steak, sliced into ¼-inch (0.5 cm) strips	625 g
⅓ cup	GF soy sauce	75 mL
1 tbsp	vegetable oil	15 mL
1	each red and yellow bell pepper, cut into ¾-inch (2 cm) cubes	1
1	medium onion, halved lengthwise, then thickly sliced	1
3	cloves garlic, minced	3
1½ tsp	minced fresh gingerroot	7 mL
3 tbsp	cornstarch	45 mL
3 tbsp	granulated sugar	45 mL
1¼ cups	GF beef stock (see Tips, left)	300 mL
3	tomatoes, cut into wedges	3
	Salt and freshly ground black pepper	
	Rice or GF pasta	

1. Place beef, in a single layer, in a shallow baking dish. Pour soy sauce over and let marinate, covered, at room temperature for 30 minutes or in the refrigerator for at least 1 hour.

2. Drain beef and discard the marinade. In a large nonstick skillet, heat oil over high heat. Stir-fry beef in two batches, for 3 minutes each time. Transfer to a plate and keep warm.

3. Reduce heat to medium. Add bell peppers, onion, garlic and gingerroot. Cook, stirring frequently, for 5 to 8 minutes or until tender-crisp.

4. In a small bowl, combine cornstarch and sugar. Whisk in beef stock. Add to skillet and cook, stirring, for 2 to 3 minutes or until thickened. Add beef and tomatoes and heat through. Season with salt and pepper to taste.

5. Spoon the stir-fry over hot rice noodles, gluten-free pasta or rice.

Meatballs for Everyday

Whether you serve these meatballs with spaghetti, sweet-and-sour sauce or as hot hors d'oeuvres, they are sure to be a hit.

VARIATIONS

Use commercial gluten-free rice crackers to make crumbs and substitute for gluten-free bread crumbs. If using flavored crackers, such as barbecue or teriyaki, omit the basil and oregano.

∾

Substitute ground turkey or chicken for all or part of the ground beef and pork.

Preheat oven to 400°F (200°C)
15-by 10-inch (40 by 25 cm) jelly roll pan, lightly greased

1 lb	extra lean ground beef	500 g
8 oz	ground pork	250 g
½ cup	finely chopped onion	125 mL
1	egg, lightly beaten	1
1 cup	soft GF bread crumbs (see Techniques Glossary, page 178)	250 mL
2 tbsp	snipped fresh parsley	25 mL
2 tbsp	snipped fresh basil leaves	25 mL
2 tbsp	snipped fresh oregano	25 mL
¼ tsp	freshly ground black pepper	1 mL

1. In a large bowl, gently mix together beef, pork, onion, egg, bread crumbs, parsley, basil, oregano and ground pepper. Shape into 1-inch (2.5 cm) balls. Place in a single layer on prepared pan.

2. Bake in a preheated oven for 20 minutes or until no longer pink in the center.

3. *To Freeze:* Cool slightly then freeze baked meatballs on the jelly roll pan. Once frozen, remove meatballs from pan and place in a heavy-duty freezer bag. Remove only the number you need — they won't stick together. Reheat meatballs from frozen directly in sauce or microwave just until thawed and then add to the sauce.

Grilled Chicken Mandarin Salad with
Sweet-and-Sour Dressing (page 24)

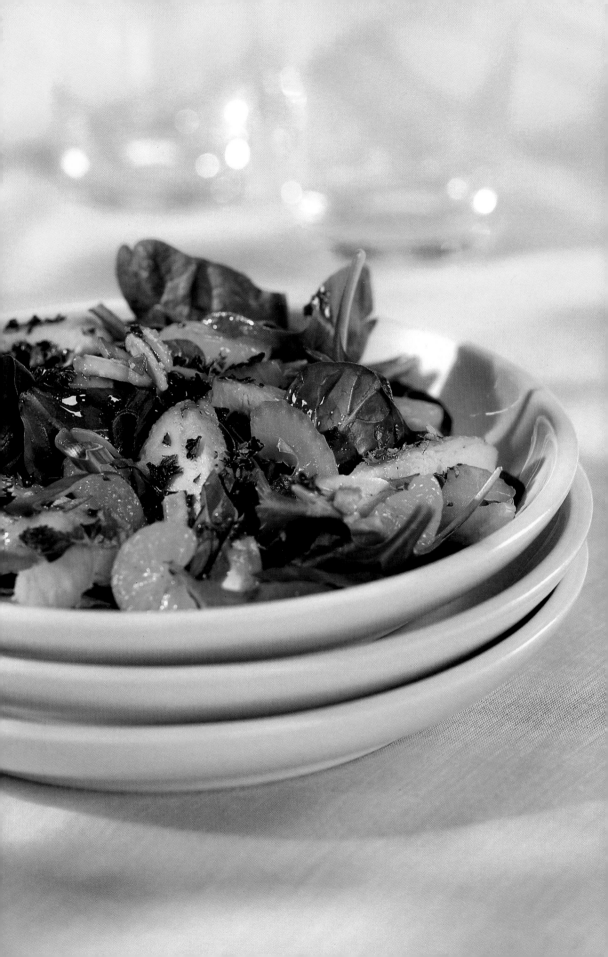

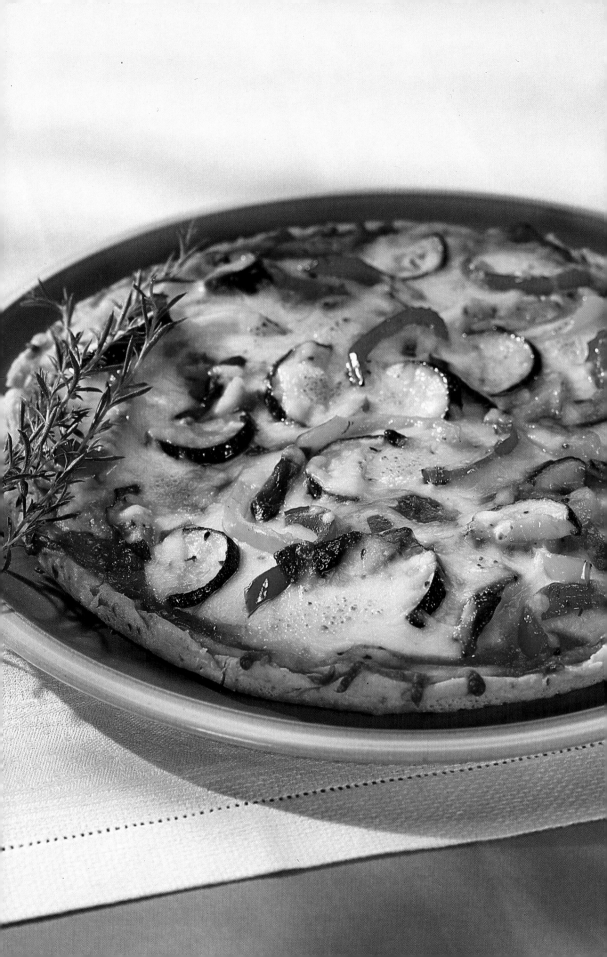

Sweet 'n' Sour Sauce

**MAKES
APPROXIMATELY
2 CUPS (500 ML)**

*Try this familiar,
not-too-sweet sauce
next time you make
Chinese food. Be sure
to include it served
over meatballs at
your next party.*

TIP
Serve this sauce over
cooked meatballs,
chicken or pork.

VARIATION
For a more colorful
sauce with a slight
tomato flavor, increase
the ketchup to
¼ cup (50 mL).

¼ cup	white vinegar	50 mL
¾ cup	water	175 mL
½ cup	packed brown sugar	125 mL
⅓ cup	granulated sugar	75 mL
2 tbsp	cornstarch	25 mL
2 tbsp	GF ketchup	25 mL
1	can (14 oz/398 mL) pineapple tidbits with juice	1

1. In a saucepan, bring vinegar, water, brown sugar and granulated sugar to a boil. Simmer gently for 2 to 3 minutes.
2. In a bowl, combine cornstarch and ketchup to form a paste. Add pineapple and juice.
3. Slowly stir pineapple mixture into the saucepan. Return to a gentle boil, stirring constantly. Simmer gently until thick and shiny.

*Thin Pizza Crust (page 50) with
Roasted Vegetable Pizza Topping (page 54)*

Barbecued Pork Sandwiches

MAKES 6 TO 8 SANDWICHES

What is better than a sloppy barbecued sandwich served outside on a hot summer day?

TIP

For faster sauce preparation, substitute 3 cups (750 mL) commercial gluten-free barbecue sauce. E-mail the manufacturer of the barbecue sauce to ask whether it is gluten-free. Many companies are pleased to send a list of gluten-free products.

SAUCE

1½ cups	GF ketchup	375 mL
1½ cups	GF chili sauce	375 mL
1 cup	water	250 mL
¼ cup	Dijon mustard	50 mL
⅓ cup	packed brown sugar	75 mL
2 tbsp	cider vinegar	25 mL
2 tsp	chili powder	10 mL
6	drops hot pepper sauce	6
6	cloves garlic, minced	6
2	large onions, diced	2

PORK

3 lbs	boneless pork shoulder or butt roast	1.5 kg
6	hamburger buns or 8 mini-sub buns (see recipe, page 36)	6

1. *Sauce:* In a saucepan, combine ketchup, chili sauce, water, Dijon mustard, brown sugar, vinegar, chili powder, hot pepper sauce, garlic and onions. Bring to a boil and simmer for 10 to 15 minutes, stirring occasionally, until thickened. Set aside to cool.

2. *Pork:* In a large glass or stainless steel bowl, pour sauce over pork roast and marinate overnight, covered, in the refrigerator.

3. Preheat barbecue to medium. Place the pork roast on a double layer of heavy-duty foil, reserving sauce. Add ½ cup (125 mL) of the sauce. Refrigerate remaining sauce. Fold foil using an envelope fold (see page 179).

VARIATIONS

VARIATIONS
Add extra diced
onions, if desired.

❧

Use a less tender cut
of beef to marinate.
Ask your butcher
for suggestions.

❧

Instead of barbecuing,
place foil-wrapped pork
in a roasting pan.
Roast at 350°F (180°C)
for approximately
2 hours or until meat
thermometer registers
160°F (70°C). Remove
cover and roast for an
extra 30 minutes.

4. Place pork roast on preheated barbecue, with lid closed, over medium coals or using indirect heat method for 1½ to 2 hours or until meat thermometer registers 160°F to 170°F (70°C to 75°C) (see Thermometers, page 172). Let roast stand for 10 to 15 minutes. Carve roast in thin slices, across the grain.

5. Meanwhile, in a saucepan, simmer remaining barbecue sauce until thickened, for at least 5 minutes. Pour sauce over sliced meat, cover and refrigerate at least 1 hour or until ready to serve. Make ahead, if you like. Then reheat in a saucepan or microwave until hot and bubbly.

6. To serve, slice each hamburger or mini-sub bun in half horizontally. On the bottom half, arrange meat slices and top with extra sauce. Top with other half of bun and press together. Serve with more sauce, if desired.

Hamburger/Mini-Sub Buns

Though formed into the traditional shape for hamburger or mini-subs, these white bread rolls make both great dinner accompaniments and sandwiches.

TIPS

If you don't have these particular shaped pans, try cast-iron corncob-shaped bread pans, English muffin rings or make free-form buns on a lightly greased baking sheet. Decrease the water by 2 tbsp (25 mL) for free-form buns.

∽

For hamburger buns, use approximately ²⁄₃ cup (150 mL) dough and for mini-sub buns ½ cup (125 mL) dough.

∽

Smooth the tops with a water-moistened rubber spatula.

Hamburger or mini-sub pans, lightly greased (see Tips, left and Equipment Glossary, page 171)

1³⁄₄ cups	rice flour	425 mL
²⁄₃ cup	potato starch	150 mL
¹⁄₃ cup	tapioca starch	75 mL
¹⁄₄ cup	non-fat dry milk or skim milk powder	50 mL
¹⁄₄ cup	granulated sugar	50 mL
2¹⁄₂ tsp	xanthan gum	12 mL
1 tbsp	bread machine or instant yeast	15 mL
1¹⁄₂ tsp	salt	7 mL
1¹⁄₄ cups	water	300 mL
1 tsp	cider vinegar	5 mL
¹⁄₄ cup	vegetable oil	50 mL
2	eggs	2
2	egg whites	2

BREAD MACHINE METHOD

1. In a large bowl or plastic bag, combine rice flour, potato starch, tapioca starch, milk powder, sugar, xanthan gum, yeast and salt. Mix well and set aside.

2. Pour water, vinegar and oil into the bread machine baking pan. Add eggs and egg whites. Select the Dough Cycle. Allow the liquids to mix until combined.

3. Gradually add the dry ingredients as the bread machine is mixing, scraping with a rubber spatula while adding. Try to incorporate all the dry ingredients within 1 to 2 minutes. Allow the bread machine to complete the cycle.

MIXER METHOD

1. In a large bowl or plastic bag, combine rice flour, potato starch, tapioca starch, milk powder, sugar, xanthan gum, yeast and salt. Mix well and set aside.

2. In a separate bowl, using a heavy-duty electric mixer with paddle attachment, combine water, vinegar, oil, eggs and egg whites until well blended.

3. With the mixer on lowest speed, slowly add the dry ingredients until combined. With a rubber spatula, scrape the bottom and sides of the bowl. With the mixer on medium speed, beat for 4 minutes.

FOR BOTH METHODS

4. Spoon into prepared pan, mounding toward the center of each individual bun (see Tips, left). Let rise in a warm, draft-free place for 30 to 45 minutes or until the dough has almost doubled in volume. Do not allow dough to over-rise. Bake in 350°F (180°C) preheated oven for 15 to 20 minutes. Remove immediately from pan to a cooling rack.

Ciabatta

From the Italian for "old slipper," ciabattas are flat, chewy loaves that are fun to make. Poke them full of dimples before rising. The flour-coated crust provides an interesting, open texture. Our round version is easily cut in wedges.

TIPS

When dusting with rice flour, use a flour sifter for a light, even sprinkle. This bread freezes well. Cut into wedges and freeze individually for sandwiches.

∾

Use English muffin rings, two-thirds full, to make individual ciabattas.

8-inch (20 cm) round baking pan, lightly floured

½ cup	whole bean flour	125 mL
½ cup	brown rice flour	125 mL
½ cup	tapioca starch	125 mL
2 tbsp	granulated sugar	25 mL
2 tsp	xanthan gum	10 mL
1 tbsp	bread machine or instant yeast	15 mL
½ tsp	salt	2 mL
¾ cup	water	175 mL
1 tsp	cider vinegar	5 mL
2 tbsp	extra virgin olive oil	25 mL
2	eggs	2
2 to 3 tbsp	sweet rice flour	25 to 45 mL

BREAD MACHINE METHOD

1. In a large bowl or plastic bag, combine whole bean flour, brown rice flour, tapioca starch, sugar, xanthan gum, yeast and salt. Mix well and set aside.

2. Pour water, vinegar and oil into the bread machine baking pan. Add eggs. Select the Dough Cycle. Allow the liquids to mix until combined.

3. Gradually add the dry ingredients as the bread machine is mixing, scraping with a rubber spatula while adding. Try to incorporate all the dry ingredients within 1 to 2 minutes. Allow the bread machine to complete the cycle.

MIXER METHOD

1. In a large bowl or plastic bag, combine the whole bean flour, brown rice flour, tapioca starch, sugar, xanthan gum, yeast and salt. Mix well and set aside.

2. In a separate bowl, using a heavy-duty electric mixer with paddle attachment, combine water, vinegar, oil and eggs until well blended.

3. With the mixer on the lowest speed, slowly add the dry ingredients until combined. With a rubber spatula, scrape the bottom and sides of the bowl. With the mixer on medium speed, beat for 4 minutes.

For a creamier-colored ciabatta, use 1 cup (250 mL) brown rice flour in place of the whole bean and brown rice flours.

FOR BOTH METHODS

4. Immediately, with a water-moistened rubber spatula, remove the sticky dough onto prepared pan. Spread evenly. Generously dust top with sweet rice flour. With well-floured fingers, make deep indents all over the dough, making sure to press all the way down to the pan. Allow to rise in a warm, draft-free place for 40 to 50 minutes or until almost double in volume. Bake in 425°F (220°C) preheated oven for 15 to 20 minutes. Remove immediately from pan to a cooling rack.

Ciabatta Sandwich Filling

MAKES 6 WEDGES

Here's a quick lunch for six adults or two teenage sons with large appetites. Our two boys devoured the whole thing between them. Try our grilled version.

TIP

Feel free to pile on lots of thinly sliced meats.

1	Ciabatta (see recipe, page 38)	1
1 to 2 tbsp	Dijon mustard	15 to 25 mL
12 oz	turkey, thinly sliced	375 g
12 oz	Swiss cheese, thinly sliced	375 g
2	large tomatoes, sliced	2
	Bean sprouts	
	Mesclun salad mix	

1. Slice baked ciabatta in half horizontally. On the bottom half, spread Dijon mustard. Arrange turkey, Swiss cheese, tomatoes, bean sprouts and mesclun greens. Top with other half of ciabatta. Cut into 6 wedges.

2. *To grill:* Brush both sides of the sandwich with a thin layer of extra virgin olive oil. Place on a hot barbecue or grill. Cook, turning once, until the sandwich is brown, crisp and the cheese is melted. Cut into wedges and serve hot. Omit Mesclun for hot sandwich.

Roast Stuffed Pork Tenderloin

SERVES 4

TIPS

To prevent the thin tip of pork tenderloin from drying, turn it under before adding the stuffing.

∾

Bread crumbs can be prepared from any gluten-free bread you prefer. Do not let dry.

Preheat oven to 350°F (180°C)
9-inch (2.5 L) square baking pan, lightly greased

¾ cup	chopped cooked broccoli	175 mL
¾ cup	soft GF bread crumbs (see Techniques Glossary, page 178)	175 mL
⅓ cup	chopped walnuts	75 mL
2 tbsp	GF chicken stock	25 mL
2 tbsp	tomato sauce	25 mL
2 tbsp	pure maple syrup	25 mL
2	pork tenderloins (each about 10 oz/300 g)	2
1 tbsp	crushed whole peppercorns	15 mL
¼ cup	tomato sauce	50 mL
¼ cup	GF chicken stock	50 mL

1. In a bowl, combine broccoli, bread crumbs, walnuts and chicken stock. Set aside.

2. In a small bowl, combine tomato sauce and maple syrup. Set aside.

3. With a sharp knife, cut tenderloins lengthwise almost in half, being careful not to cut all the way through. Open and flatten to butterfly. If still too thick, cut the thicker piece again, being careful to leave the tenderloin in one piece. Spoon half the broccoli stuffing over each of the tenderloins.

VARIATION

Short on time? No need
to roll and tie the pork
loin. After topping
with stuffing, bake,
stuffing-side up, in
preheated oven for
20 to 30 minutes.

4. Starting at one long side, roll each tenderloin like a jelly roll and tie tightly with string. Roll in tomato-maple syrup mixture, then in crushed peppercorns. Place in prepared baking dish and bake in a preheated oven for 30 to 45 minutes or until meat thermometer registers 160°F (70°C) or a hint of pink remains in pork. Remove tenderloins and let stand for 5 minutes, covered lightly with foil to keep warm.

5. For the sauce, add tomato sauce and chicken stock to pan drippings. Stir and cook over medium heat until hot and bubbly. Pour sauce onto individual serving plates. Remove string. Slice tenderloins and place on top of sauce.

Chicken Cacciatore

SERVES 6 TO 8

Italian for "hunter-style," this dish is perfect to put in the slow cooker for weeknights when family members must eat at different times. It's even tastier the next day!

TIP
Boneless chicken breasts make this special when serving guests.

VARIATIONS
Use a whole chicken, skinned and cut into pieces, in place of the breasts.

∾

Add raw shrimp in addition to or instead of the chicken. Add shrimp during the last 30 minutes of cooking.

4-quart (4 L) slow cooker

4	large bell peppers, assorted colors, cut into ½-inch (1 cm) strips	4
2	medium onions, thickly sliced	2
8 oz	large mushrooms, thickly sliced	250 g
8	skinless, bone-in chicken breasts (see Tip, left)	8
2 cups	GF pasta sauce	500 mL
¼ cup	dry red wine (optional)	50 mL
	Rice or GF pasta	

1. Place peppers, onions, mushrooms, chicken and pasta sauce in the slow cooker stoneware. Cook on High for 4 hours or on Low for 6 hours or until chicken is tender. If desired, add red wine during the last 30 minutes. Serve over rice or gluten-free pasta.

Crunchy Almond Chicken

SERVES 6

Need a quick main dish for dinner? Sprinkle extra almonds on the pan to toast as the chicken bakes.

TIP

The chicken is cooked when an instant read thermometer registers 170°F (75°C).

VARIATIONS

Use commercial gluten-free rice crackers to make crumbs or substitute for gluten-free bread crumbs.

༄

Substitute basil, marjoram or thyme for the rosemary.

༄

Substitute boneless fish fillets for the chicken.

Preheat oven to 350°F (180°C)
15-by 10-inch (40 by 25 cm) jelly roll pan, lightly greased

⅓ cup	plain yogurt	75 mL
¼ cup	Dijon mustard	50 mL
½ cup	soft GF bread crumbs (see Techniques Glossary, page 178)	125 mL
⅓ cup	sliced almonds	75 mL
1 tsp	dried rosemary	5 mL
½ tsp	salt	2 mL
¼ tsp	freshly ground black pepper	1 mL
6	skinless, boneless chicken breasts	6

1. On a pie plate, combine yogurt and Dijon mustard. Set aside. On a second pie plate, combine bread crumbs, almonds, rosemary, salt and pepper.

2. Roll chicken first in yogurt-mustard mixture and then in the seasoned bread crumbs.

3. Place in a single layer on prepared pan. Bake in a preheated oven for 30 to 35 minutes or until golden brown and chicken juice runs clear.

Chicken Pot Pie

> *Crave Grandma's country cooking? Take pleasure in the aroma of the chicken simmering when you're home during the weekend.*

TIPS

For a more flavorful stock, use bone-in chicken. If available, add a couple of backs and necks.

∽

If only boneless chicken pieces are available, purchase 2 lbs (1 kg) and add at least 2 to 3 tsp (10 to 15 mL) gluten-free chicken stock powder.

∽

Freeze any leftover stock to use in other recipes.

∽

Make stock in the slow cooker — just leave it on all day. Refrigerating the stock overnight makes it easier to remove any fat that has risen to the surface.

8-cup (2 L) shallow casserole

STOCK

2½ lbs	whole chicken or bone-in chicken pieces	1.25 kg
1	carrot, coarsely chopped	1
1	medium onion, thickly sliced	1
8	peppercorns	8
1	bay leaf	1
3 cups	water	750 mL

STEW

1 cup	green beans, cut into 1-inch (2.5 cm) pieces	250 mL
1 cup	baby carrots, cut in half	250 mL
2	medium potatoes, cut into ½-inch (1 cm) cubes	2
1	stalk celery, sliced	1
⅓ cup	cornstarch	75 mL
1 cup	milk	250 mL
2 tsp	dried thyme leaves	10 mL
4 cups	reserved stock from chicken	1 L
	Salt and freshly ground black pepper to taste	
½	Pie Pastry (see recipe, page 136)	½

1. *Stock:* In a large saucepan, combine chicken, carrot, onion, peppercorns, bay leaf and water. Bring to a boil. Then skim off froth. Reduce heat, cover, and simmer for 60 minutes or until chicken is tender.

2. Strain, reserving stock. Discard carrot, onion, peppercorns and bay leaf. Cut chicken into large chunks. Skim fat off stock.

Make 4 to 6 individual pot pies, then freeze them. To serve, bake from frozen until hot and bubbly or a meat thermometer registers 175°F (80°C).

3. *Stew:* In a steamer or microwave, steam green beans, carrots, potatoes and celery just until tender. Set aside.

4. In a large saucepan, combine cornstarch, milk, thyme and 4 cups (1 L) reserved stock. Cook, stirring constantly, until mixture boils and thickens. Add chicken and vegetables. Spoon stew into the casserole.

5. Roll out pastry. Place on stew and cut steam vents. Bake in a 400°F (200°C) preheated oven for 25 to 35 minutes or until hot and bubbly.

Santa Fe Chicken

SERVES 4 TO 6

Fire-roasted vegetables and strips of chicken breast over gluten-free pasta — no wonder it is a top seller in many restaurants.

TIPS

Cook gluten-free pasta just until al dente.

❧

This recipe can easily be halved to serve two.

❧

Roast extra vegetables to serve another day.

VARIATIONS

Substitute chunks of cooked pork or beef for the chicken.

❧

For a spicier dish, substitute a hot pepper for one of the bell peppers.

❧

To speed up the preparation, use a packaged mix of stir-fry vegetables instead of roasting the vegetables. Steam just until tender before adding.

Preheat oven 425°F (220°C)
Roasting pan

1 tbsp	extra virgin olive oil	15 mL
1	small Italian eggplant, cut into 1-inch (2.5 cm) cubes	1
1	large red or yellow bell pepper, cut into 1-inch (2.5 cm) strips	1
3 cups	Portobello mushrooms, cut into ½-inch (1 cm) thick slices	750 mL
2	small zucchini, cut into ½-inch (1 cm) slices	2
6	cloves garlic, minced	6
8 to 12 oz	GF rice fettuccine or GF rotini pasta	250 to 375 g
¼ cup	butter	50 mL
1	can (14 oz/385 mL) evaporated milk	1
½ cup	freshly grated Parmesan cheese	125 mL
⅓ cup	snipped fresh cilantro	75 mL
2	cooked skinless, boneless chicken breasts, cut into 1-inch (2.5 cm) strips	2
1	can (19 oz/540 mL) black beans, rinsed and drained	1
1 tbsp	freshly squeezed lime juice	15 mL
¾ cup	shredded Monterey Jack cheese	175 mL

1. Measure oil into roasting pan. Add vegetables and garlic and toss to coat. Roast in preheated oven, turning once, for 10 to 15 minutes or until tender. Do not overcook. Set aside to cool.

2. In a large pot of boiling water, cook pasta according to package directions. Drain but do not rinse.

3. In a large saucepan, combine pasta, butter, evaporated milk, Parmesan cheese and cilantro. Cook over medium heat, stirring constantly, until hot and bubbly. Add roasted vegetables, chicken, black beans and lime juice. Heat until steaming.

4. Spoon into large serving bowl and top with cheese.

Turkey Meat Loaf

SERVES 4 TO 6

Microwave-safe 9-inch (23 cm) ring mold, ungreased

> *Quick, easy and always popular, this meat loaf is great served with boiled new potatoes and fresh green beans.*

1½ lbs	extra lean ground turkey	750 g
½ cup	tomato sauce	125 mL
⅓ cup	soft GF bread crumbs (see Techniques Glossary, page 178)	75 mL
¼ cup	rice bran	50 mL
¼ cup	finely chopped onion	50 mL
1	egg, lightly beaten	1
½ tsp	salt	2 mL
¼ tsp	freshly ground black pepper	1 mL
	Mustard Sauce (see recipe, below)	

TIP

For a conventional meat loaf, top with Mustard Sauce, then bake in an ungreased 9-by 5-inch (2 L) loaf pan in a 350°F (180°C) oven for 35 to 45 minutes.

VARIATION

Substitute ground beef, veal, chicken or a combination for the ground turkey.

1. In a bowl, gently mix together turkey, tomato sauce, bread crumbs, rice bran, onion, egg, salt and pepper.
2. Spoon into mold and cover with waxed paper. Microwave on High for 10 minutes or until partially set. Drain.
3. Spoon Mustard Sauce over meat loaf. Microwave on High for 2 to 3 minutes or until meat thermometer registers 175°F (80°C).
4. Let stand covered with foil for 5 minutes before serving.

Mustard Sauce

MAKES ⅔ CUP (150 ML)

> *Cousin George loves to serve this slightly tangy sauce to complement meatballs, pork chops and veal.*

½ cup	tomato sauce	125 mL
2 tbsp	packed brown sugar	25 mL
2 tbsp	freshly squeezed lemon juice	25 mL
1 tbsp	prepared mustard	15 mL

1. In a small bowl, combine tomato sauce, brown sugar, lemon juice and mustard.

Plain Pizza Crust

MAKES 1 CRUST

For a traditional pizza crust, try this recipe.

TIPS

This recipe can be easily doubled to make two pizza crusts. Partially bake both, top one to bake and eat. Freeze the other to use later.

～

Warming the finished pizza for 5 minutes in the oven results in a very crisp crust.

～

Use as much sweet rice flour as you need to handle the dough. It is tasteless in the baked crust. You need less and less, the more you perfect this technique.

One 12-inch (30 cm) pizza pan, generously greased

¾ cup	brown rice flour	175 mL
⅓ cup	potato starch	75 mL
1 tsp	granulated sugar	5 mL
1½ tsp	xanthan gum	7 mL
1½ tsp	bread machine or instant yeast	7 mL
½ tsp	salt	2 mL
1 tsp	dried oregano leaves	5 mL
¾ cup	water	175 mL
1 tsp	cider vinegar	5 mL
1 tbsp	vegetable oil	15 mL
2 to 3 tbsp	sweet rice flour	25 to 45 mL

BREAD MACHINE METHOD

1. In a large bowl or plastic bag, combine brown rice flour, potato starch, sugar, xanthan gum, yeast, salt and oregano. Mix well and set aside.

2. Pour water, vinegar and oil into the bread machine baking pan. Select the Dough Cycle. Allow the liquids to mix until combined.

3. Gradually add the dry ingredients as the bread machine is mixing, scraping with a rubber spatula while adding. Try to incorporate all the dry ingredients within 1 to 2 minutes. Allow the bread machine to complete the cycle.

VARIATION
Substitute your favorite
herb for the oregano
— try basil, marjoram
or thyme.

MIXER METHOD

1. In a large bowl or plastic bag, combine brown rice flour, potato starch, sugar, xanthan gum, yeast, salt and oregano. Mix well and set aside.

2. In a separate bowl, using a heavy-duty electric mixer with paddle attachment, combine water, vinegar and oil until well blended.

3. With the mixer on the lowest speed, slowly add the dry ingredients until combined. With a rubber spatula, scrape the bottom and sides of the bowl. With the mixer on medium speed, beat for 4 minutes.

FOR BOTH METHODS

4. With a wet rubber spatula, remove the very sticky dough to prepared pan, spreading out as much as possible. Generously sprinkle with sweet rice flour. With floured fingers, gently pat out dough to fill the pan evenly. Continue to sprinkle with sweet rice flour as required. Form a rim at the edge of pan. Allow to rise in a warm, draft-free place for 15 minutes. Bake in 400°F (200°C) preheated oven for 12 to 15 minutes or until firm. Spread with your choice of toppings (see recipes, pages 52 to 54). Return to oven and bake according to recipe topping directions.

Thin Pizza Crust

MAKES 2 CRUSTS

Two 12-inch (30 cm) pizza pans, lightly greased

> *Try our version of right-to-the-edge thin crust pizza.*

TIPS

This dough is thin enough to pour onto the pizza pans. It can be quickly spread to the edges with a moist rubber spatula.

∽

Don't worry about the cracks on the surface of this crust after 10 minutes of baking. Expect slight shrinkage from the edges.

1 cup	whole bean flour	250 mL
1 cup	sorghum flour	250 mL
1/3 cup	tapioca starch	75 mL
1 tsp	granulated sugar	5 mL
1/2 tsp	xanthan gum	2 mL
1 1/2 tsp	bread machine or instant yeast	7 mL
1 tsp	salt	5 mL
1 tsp	dried oregano leaves	5 mL
1 3/4 cups	water	425 mL
1 tsp	cider vinegar	5 mL
2 tbsp	vegetable oil	25 mL

BREAD MACHINE METHOD

1. In a large bowl or plastic bag, combine whole bean flour, sorghum flour, tapioca starch, sugar, xanthan gum, yeast, salt and oregano. Mix well and set aside.

2. Pour water, vinegar and oil into the bread machine baking pan. Select the Dough Cycle.

3. Gradually add the dry ingredients as the bread machine is mixing, scraping with a rubber spatula while adding. Try to incorporate all the dry ingredients within 1 to 2 minutes. Allow the bread machine to complete the cycle.

VARIATIONS

This dough can be divided into equal portions to make eight 6-inch (15 cm) individual pizzas. Bake on greased baking sheets for 10 to 12 minutes.

❧

Use 1 tbsp (15 mL) chopped fresh oregano for the dried herb.

MIXER METHOD

1. In a large bowl or plastic bag, combine whole bean flour, sorghum flour, tapioca starch, sugar, xanthan gum, yeast, salt and oregano. Mix well and set aside.

2. In a separate bowl, using a heavy-duty electric mixer with paddle attachment, combine water, vinegar and oil until well blended.

3. With the mixer on the lowest speed, slowly add the dry ingredients until combined. With a rubber spatula, scrape the bottom and sides of the bowl. With the mixer on medium speed, beat for 4 minutes.

FOR BOTH METHODS

4. Immediately pour onto prepared pans. Spread evenly with a water-moistened rubber spatula. Allow to rise in a warm, draft-free place for 15 minutes. Bake in 400°F (200°C) preheated oven for 12 to 15 minutes or until firm. Spread with your choice of toppings (see recipes, pages 52 to 54). Return to oven and bake according to recipe topping directions.

Leek-Mushroom Pizza Topping

MAKES TOPPING FOR ONE 12-INCH (30 CM) PIZZA

Subtle leeks blend the flavors of mushrooms and pesto.

VARIATIONS

Substitute extra Parmesan for the Asiago to make a totally Parmesan cheese topping.

∾

Strips of cooked chicken can be added to the leek-mushroom mixture before adding the cheeses.

∾

Substitute a commercial pesto sauce for the homemade.

Preheat oven to 400°F (200°C)

1 tbsp	extra virgin olive oil	15 mL
2	leeks, sliced in half lengthwise, then cut into $\frac{1}{2}$-inch (1 cm) pieces, white and light green parts only	2
2 cups	cremini mushroom caps, halved then sliced into $\frac{1}{2}$-inch (1 cm) pieces	500 mL
$\frac{1}{3}$ cup	Parsley Pesto Sauce (see recipe, 53)	75 mL
$\frac{2}{3}$ cup	freshly grated Asiago cheese	150 mL
$\frac{1}{3}$ cup	freshly grated Parmesan cheese	75 mL
1	partially baked pizza crust (see recipes, pages 48 and 50)	1

1. In a frying pan, heat oil over medium-high heat. Add leeks and mushrooms and sauté, stirring constantly, until tender, about 3 to 5 minutes. Set aside.

2. Spread pesto over pizza crust. Top with leek-mushroom mixture, then Asiago and Parmesan cheese.

3. Bake the regular-size pizza in a preheated oven for 15 to 20 minutes or smaller pizzas for 10 to 12 minutes or until cheese is lightly browned and heated through.

Parsley Pesto Sauce

MAKES ⅔ CUP (150 ML)

When fresh basil is plentiful, make lots of sauce and freeze to use in the winter.

2	large cloves garlic	2
1 cup	fresh parsley leaves, tightly packed	250 mL
⅓ cup	fresh basil leaves, tightly packed	75 mL
1 tbsp	extra virgin olive oil	15 mL
¼ cup	freshly grated Parmesan cheese	50 mL
¼ cup	GF vegetable stock	50 mL

1. In a food processor, with processor on, drop garlic through the tube and process until chopped. Add basil, parsley, oil and Parmesan cheese. Process until well mixed. With a rubber spatula, scrape the sides once or twice. Add stock, process until well blended.

Five-Cheese Pizza Topping

MAKES TOPPING FOR ONE 12-INCH (30 CM) PIZZA

We love cheese and couldn't decide which we like the best on pizza — so we mixed five together. Which five do you like?

TIP
Check for gluten before you purchase a packaged shredded cheese mix.

VARIATION
Use tomato or gluten-free pizza sauce for the salsa.

Preheat oven to 400°F (200°C)

1 to 2 oz	freshly grated Asiago cheese	30 to 60 g
1 to 2 oz	shredded old Cheddar cheese	30 to 60 g
1 to 2 oz	shredded Fontina cheese	30 to 60 g
1 to 2 oz	crumbled Gorgonzola cheese	30 to 60 g
1 to 2 oz	shredded Havarti cheese	30 to 60 g
1 cup	chunky salsa	250 mL
1	partially baked pizza crust (see recipes, page 48 and 50)	1

1. In a small bowl, mix together cheeses. Set aside.
2. Spread salsa over pizza crust, then top with cheese mixture.
3. Bake in preheated oven for 15 to 20 minutes or until cheese is lightly browned and heated through.

Roasted Vegetable Pizza Topping

MAKES TOPPING FOR ONE 12-INCH (30 CM) PIZZA

Like lots of topping with every bite of pizza? Try our simplified version — thin, edgeless and filled to the brim!

TIP
We like to sprinkle some of the cheese on the crust before topping as this helps the vegetables remain on the pizza.

VARIATION
For a stronger cheese combination, try Asiago and Romano.

Preheat oven to 425°F (220°C)
Roasting pan

1 tbsp	extra virgin olive oil	15 mL
2	small Italian eggplants, cut into ½-inch (1 cm) cubes	2
1	large red bell pepper, cut into ½-inch (1 cm) slices	1
1	large yellow bell pepper, cut into ½-inch (1 cm) slices	1
3 cups	Portobello mushrooms, cut into ½-inch (1 cm) thick slices, about 10 oz (300 g)	750 mL
4	small zucchini, cut into ½-inch (1 cm) slices	4
6	cloves garlic, minced	6
⅔ cup	shredded mozzarella cheese	150 mL
½ cup	freshly grated Parmesan cheese	125 mL
1	partially baked pizza crust (see recipes, pages 48 and 50)	1

1. Measure oil into roasting pan. Add vegetables and garlic. Toss to coat. Roast in preheated oven, turning once, for 10 to 15 minutes or until tender. Do not overcook. Set aside to cool.

2. To assemble, sprinkle half the mozzarella cheese over the partially baked pizza crust. Top with roasted vegetables, remaining mozzarella and Parmesan. Reduce heat to 400°F (200°C) and bake for 12 to 15 minutes or until the topping is bubbly and cheese is melted, lightly browned and heated through. Serve immediately.

Scalloped Potatoes with a New Twist

SERVES 4 TO 6

An old-fashioned comfort food updated for today. If you can't tolerate dairy products, it's a bonus.

TIPS

Use the slicing blade of a food processor to slice potatoes thinly.

∾

Dark green leaves of celery are most flavorful.

∾

If the gluten-free chicken stock powder is unsalted, season with salt to taste.

VARIATION

For a potluck dish, double or triple the recipe and use a 20- to 30-cup (5 to 7.5 L) casserole and increase the baking time by 15 to 30 minutes or until fork-tender.

Preheat oven to 350°F (180°C)
10-cup (2.5 L) casserole

1	medium onion, diced	1
½ cup	celery leaves	125 mL
3 tbsp	butter or margarine	45 mL
2 tbsp	potato starch	25 mL
2 tbsp	GF chicken stock powder	25 mL
3 to 4 cups	water	750 mL to 1 L
¼ tsp	freshly ground black pepper	1 mL
2 lbs	potatoes, thinly sliced	1 kg

1. In a food processor, combine onion, celery leaves, butter, potato starch, chicken stock powder, 3 cups (750 mL) water and ground pepper until combined. Set aside.

2. In casserole, spread potatoes evenly. Pour sauce over top. If necessary, add extra water so potatoes are almost covered. The amount depends on the size and shape of the casserole.

3. Bake, uncovered, in preheated oven for 75 to 90 minutes or until potatoes are fork-tender.

Vegetable Cobbler

SERVES 4 TO 6

> A recipe that originated in Romania inspired this drop biscuit-topped vegetable casserole. Although not a cobbler in the traditional sense, it is every bit as comforting.

TIPS

To help preserve the vegetables' bright color, don't lift the lid while they are cooking.

❧

Have the cobbler topping ready to drop on the vegetables as soon as they are cooked.

❧

Be sure not to overcook the vegetables in Step 3. They will continue to cook as the biscuits bake.

❧

See Biscuits and Cobblers, page 62.

Preheat oven to 350°F (180°C)
Deep 12-cup (3 L) covered casserole

1½ cups	winter squash, peeled and cut into 1-inch (2.5 cm) cubes	375 mL
1 cup	green beans, cut into 1½-inch (4 cm) pieces	250 mL
2	medium carrots, cut into ½-inch (1 cm) thick slices	2
1	stalk celery, cut into ½-inch (1 cm) thick slices	1
½	large red bell pepper, cut into ¾-inch (2 cm) strips	½
1	medium zucchini, cut into ½-inch (1 cm) pieces	1
3	cloves garlic, minced	3
1	bay leaf	1
½ cup	GF chicken, beef or vegetable stock	125 mL
½ cup	water	125 mL
2 tbsp	extra virgin olive oil	25 mL
1 tsp	salt	5 mL
1 tsp	dried tarragon leaves	5 mL
2	medium tomatoes, quartered	2
	Cobbler Biscuit (see recipe, page 57)	

1. In casserole dish, mix together squash, beans, carrots, celery, bell pepper, zucchini, garlic and bay leaf. Set aside.

2. In a small bowl, combine stock, water, oil, salt and tarragon. Microwave on High for 2 to 4 minutes or heat in saucepan over medium heat until hot and bubbly. Pour stock mixture over vegetables.

3. Bake, covered, in preheated oven for 30 to 40 minutes or until vegetables are slightly crisp. Do not overcook. Meanwhile, prepare the Cobbler Biscuit.

Choose other vegetables you like such as parsnips, turnip, sweet potatoes, cauliflower, broccoli, eggplant and cabbage. Soft vegetables should be left in larger pieces so they cook in the same time as the harder vegetables.

∾

Substitute fresh or dry herbs for the tarragon.

COBBLER BISCUIT

1 cup	whole bean flour	250 mL
¼ cup	tapioca starch	50 mL
1 tbsp	granulated sugar	15 mL
1 tsp	xanthan gum	5 mL
1½ tsp	GF baking powder	7 mL
½ tsp	baking soda	2 mL
¼ tsp	salt	1 mL
¼ cup	shortening	50 mL
1 cup	buttermilk	250 mL

1. In a large bowl, stir together whole bean flour, tapioca starch, sugar, xanthan gum, baking powder, baking soda and salt.

2. Using a pastry blender or two knives, cut in shortening until mixture resembles coarse crumbs. Add buttermilk all at once, stirring with a fork to make very sticky dough. Let stand for up to 30 minutes.

3. Remove vegetables from oven. Quickly stir the tomatoes into the casserole. Drop prepared biscuit topping, by heaping tablespoonfuls (15 mL), onto hot bubbly vegetable mixture.

4. Increase oven temperature to 425°F (220°C). Bake for 15 to 20 minutes or until biscuits are browned. Serve immediately.

Tempura

> Today, we think of tempura to describe a light, crispy batter. Perfect for vegetables as well as seafood.

TIPS

Don't omit the cayenne pepper — it helps the batter to brown.

∾

If the cayenne is too hot for your taste buds, you can also use paprika (see Variations, below).

VARIATIONS

Substitute ¼ tsp (1 mL) paprika for the cayenne pepper. Paprika also helps the batter to brown as it cooks.

∾

Use whitefish fillets and any vegetable combination.

Preheat oil in deep fryer or wok to 350°F (180°C)

1 cup	potato starch	250 mL
2 tsp	GF baking powder	10 mL
½ tsp	salt	2 mL
⅛ tsp	cayenne pepper (see Tips, left)	0.5 mL
¾ cup	milk	175 mL
1 tbsp	vegetable oil	15 mL
1	egg	1
½ cup	sweet rice flour	125 mL
	Vegetable oil for frying	
1 lb	large shrimp, peeled and deveined	500 g
1 lb	large scallops	500 g
1	sweet potato, cut into ⅛-inch (0.25 cm) slices	1
2	small zucchini, cut into ¼-inch (0.5 cm) slices	2
4 oz	button mushrooms	125 g
4	green onions, cut into 1-inch (2.5 cm) pieces	4

1. In a large bowl or plastic bag, combine potato starch, baking powder, salt and cayenne pepper. Mix well and set aside.

2. In a separate bowl, using an electric mixer, combine the milk, oil and egg. With the mixer on the lowest speed, slowly add the dry ingredients until combined. With a rubber spatula, scrape the bottom and sides of the bowl.

3. Dredge seafood and vegetables in sweet rice flour. Dip a few pieces at a time into prepared batter to generously coat.

4. Deep-fry until golden. Drain on paper towels. Serve immediately.

Batter-Fried Fish

SERVES 4

*The crisp, light batter
satisfies the craving
for fish and chips.
Treat yourself.*

TIP
Don't omit the paprika
— it helps the batter to
lightly brown.

VARIATION
For a spicier coating,
substitute a pinch
of cayenne pepper
for the paprika.

Preheat oil in deep fryer or wok to 350°F (180°C)

2	egg whites	2
⅓ cup	cornstarch	75 mL
½ tsp	paprika	2 mL
1 lb	fish fillets, such as sole, haddock or tilapia	500 g
¼ cup	sweet rice flour	50 mL
	Vegetable oil for frying	

1. In a small bowl, using an electric mixer, beat egg whites until stiff but not dry. Sift cornstarch and paprika over beaten egg whites. With a rubber spatula, fold in. Set aside.

2. Rinse fillets under cold running water and pat dry. Dredge in sweet rice flour. Dip into prepared batter to generously coat, leaving as much batter on the fish as possible.

3. Deep-fry fish for 2 to 4 minutes on each side or until coating is crisp and the fish is fork-tender. Drain on paper towels.

Seafood Lasagna

SERVES 6 TO 8

This is another example of a dish adopted by North Americans that has become a staple of our diet — enjoy our seafood version.

TIPS

Use any combination of your favorite seafood — choose from scallops, shrimp, whitefish, crab, lobster, clams or oysters.

∽

A 6-oz (175 g) package of baby spinach contains approximately 3 cups (750 mL).

∽

Purchase 7 oz (200 g) shredded mozzarella cheese.

∽

Freeze leftover lasagna in individual amounts. Thaw and reheat in the microwave.

VARIATION

Use 1 lb (500 g) ground beef or chicken instead of the seafood. Cook the meat before sautéeing the vegetables.

Preheat oven to 350°F (180°C)
13-by 9-inch (3 L) baking pan

9	GF rice lasagna noodles	9
2 tsp	extra virgin olive oil	10 mL
1	red or yellow bell pepper, diced	1
1	medium onion, diced	1
1	jar (25 oz/700 mL) GF pasta sauce	1
2 tbsp	dry white wine (optional)	25 mL
1½ lbs	cooked seafood (see Tips, left)	750 g
1 cup	cottage cheese	250 mL
1	egg, slightly beaten	1
6 oz	baby spinach, washed and dried	175 g
2 cups	shredded mozzarella cheese	500 mL
½ cup	freshly grated Parmesan cheese	125 mL

1. In a large pot of gently boiling water, cook lasagna noodles according to package directions. Drain, rinse well with cold water, then set aside.

2. In a saucepan, heat oil over medium-high heat. Add bell pepper and onion. Sauté until tender. Add pasta sauce and simmer for 5 to 10 minutes or until hot and bubbly. Add wine, if using, then set aside.

3. In a small bowl, combine cottage cheese and egg. Set aside.

4. To assemble, spread a thin layer of pasta sauce mixture in baking pan. Top with 3 lasagna noodles. Cover with one-third of remaining pasta sauce, half the spinach, half the cottage cheese mixture, half the seafood and sprinkle with half the mozzarella cheese.

5. Cover with 3 lasagna noodles and repeat layering with half the remaining pasta sauce, the remaining spinach, cottage cheese mixture, seafood and mozzarella cheese. Cover with the remaining lasagna noodles, pasta sauce and Parmesan cheese.

6. Bake in preheated oven for 40 to 50 minutes or until bubbly and cheese is golden brown. Let stand 10 to 15 minutes before serving.

Quick Breads

*Perfect for breakfast, lunch or a portable snack,
quick breads are full of flavor. Enjoy muffins and
biscuits hot from the oven. Keep several in the freezer.*

~ Quick Bread ~
Baking Tips

- Gluten-free muffin and quick bread loaf batters should be the same consistency as wheat flour batters; however, you can mix gluten-free batters more without producing tough products that are full of holes.

- Fill muffin cups level with the top and loaf pans no more than three-quarters full. Let the batter stand for 30 minutes. The resulting texture is worth the wait, as it is more tender. If you are short of time bake immediately.

- If the baked muffins stick to the lightly greased muffin tin cups, let them stand a few minutes (but not too long) after removing them from the oven. If allowed to stay in the pan too long, the muffins become soggy. If muffins stick, loosen gently with a spatula.

- Wrap muffins and quick bread loaves while still warm to prevent them from drying too quickly. Wrap individual muffins or quick bread slices, then place several in a larger airtight plastic bag to freeze. Pack frozen in your lunch box to thaw in time for a mid-morning snack.

~ Biscuits and Cobblers ~

- Shortening or cold butter is cut into the dry ingredients with a pastry blender just until it resembles coarse cornmeal or pieces the size of small peas. Cold butter cuts in more quickly when pre-cut into 1-inch (2.5 cm) cubes.

- Fill lightly greased English muffin rings about two-thirds full. Smooth the top slightly for more traditional biscuits. The easiest way to grease English muffin rings (see Equipment Glossary, page 171) is to place them on a baking sheet then spray the sheet and the rings at the same time.

- Make only a few biscuits at a time. They are at their best served warm from the oven. Reheat for just a few seconds in the microwave.

- Cobbler toppings are a drop biscuit. The fruit or vegetable bases must be boiling and piping hot before the topping is spooned on. The bottom of the biscuit cooks from the heat of the bubbling liquid. If the base is cold, the center and bottom of the biscuit may be gummy when the top is browned and baked.

- Leave space between the biscuits for the hot liquid to bubble up, preventing them from boiling over.

Applesauce Raisin Muffins

MAKES 12 MUFFINS

Here's a truly "everything free" muffin — gluten-free, fat-free and yeast-free — everything except sweetness and flavor!

TIP

If sweetened applesauce is used, decrease the granulated sugar to ⅓ cup (75 mL).

VARIATIONS

Substitute an equal amount of prune purée for the applesauce.

Spoon batter into a lightly greased 9-by 5-inch (2 L) loaf pan and bake 65 to 75 minutes or until a cake tester inserted in the center comes out clean.

Preheat oven to 350°F (180°C)
Muffin tin, lightly greased

1⅓ cups	sorghum flour	325 mL
⅓ cup	whole bean flour	75 mL
⅓ cup	cornstarch	75 mL
½ cup	granulated sugar	125 mL
2 tsp	xanthan gum	10 mL
1 tsp	GF baking powder	5 mL
½ tsp	baking soda	2 mL
¼ tsp	salt	1 mL
½ tsp	ground cinnamon	2 mL
1 cup	raisins	250 mL
1½ cups	unsweetened applesauce (see Tip, left)	375 mL
1 tsp	cider vinegar	5 mL
2	egg whites	2

1. In a large bowl, stir together sorghum flour, whole bean flour, cornstarch, sugar, xanthan gum, baking powder, baking soda, salt, cinnamon and raisins. Set aside.

2. In a separate bowl, using an electric mixer or whisk, beat applesauce, vinegar and egg whites until combined.

3. Pour applesauce mixture over dry ingredients and stir just until combined. Spoon into each cup of prepared muffin tin. Let stand for 30 minutes.

4. Bake in preheated oven for 20 to 25 minutes or until firm to the touch. Remove from the pan immediately and let cool completely on a rack.

Banana Nut Muffins

MAKES 12 MUFFINS

> *With all the same great moist banana flavor of traditional Banana Nut Bread, this gluten-free muffin is sure to please.*

TIPS

Stir the dry ingredients thoroughly before adding to the liquids. The rice flour and starches are so finely textured, they clump very easily.

∽

If muffins stick to the pan, let stand for 2 to 3 minutes before trying again to remove them.

VARIATIONS

Substitute pecans or ⅓ cup (75 mL) slightly cracked flaxseed for the walnuts.

∽

For traditional Banana Bread, omit the walnuts and spoon the batter into a lightly greased 9-by 5-inch (2 L) loaf pan. Bake at 325°F (160°C) for 50 to 60 minutes or until a cake tester inserted in the center comes out clean.

Preheat oven to 350°F (180°C)
Muffin tin, lightly greased

1¼ cups	brown rice flour	300 mL
½ cup	potato starch	125 mL
¼ cup	tapioca starch	50 mL
½ tsp	xanthan gum	2 mL
1 tsp	GF baking powder	5 mL
1 tsp	baking soda	5 mL
¼ tsp	salt	1 mL
¾ cup	chopped walnuts	175 mL
1⅓ cups	mashed banana	325 mL
1 tsp	cider vinegar	5 mL
¼ cup	vegetable oil	50 mL
2	eggs	2
¼ cup	liquid honey	50 mL

1. In a large bowl, stir together rice flour, potato starch, tapioca starch, xanthan gum, baking powder, baking soda, salt and walnuts. Set aside.

2. In a separate bowl, using an electric mixer, beat banana, vinegar, oil and eggs until combined. Add honey while mixing.

3. Pour banana mixture over dry ingredients and stir just until combined. Spoon into each cup of prepared muffin tin. Let stand for 30 minutes.

4. Bake in preheated oven for 15 to 20 minutes or until firm to the touch. Remove from the pan immediately and let cool completely on a rack.

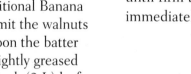

Batter-Fried Fish (page 59)

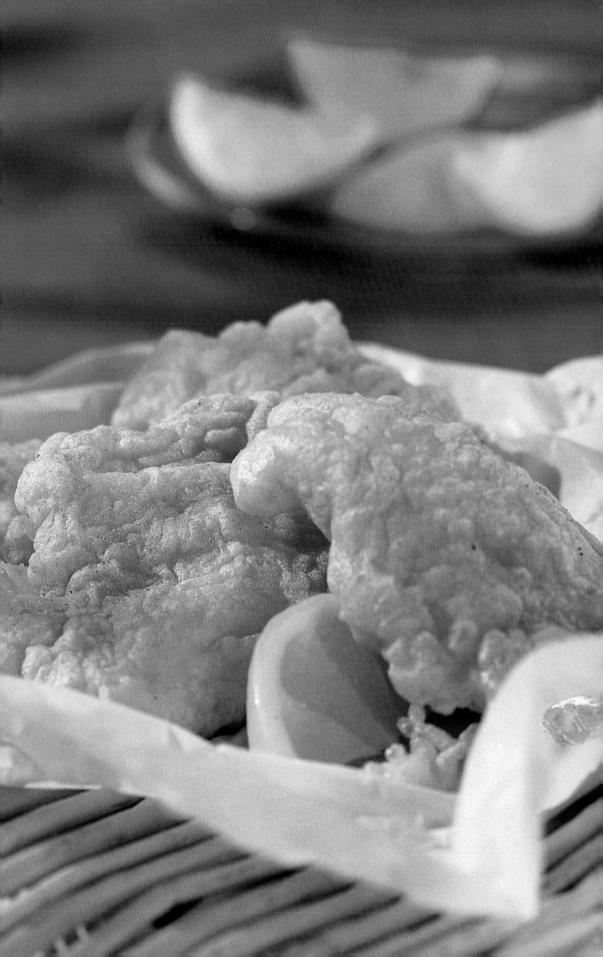

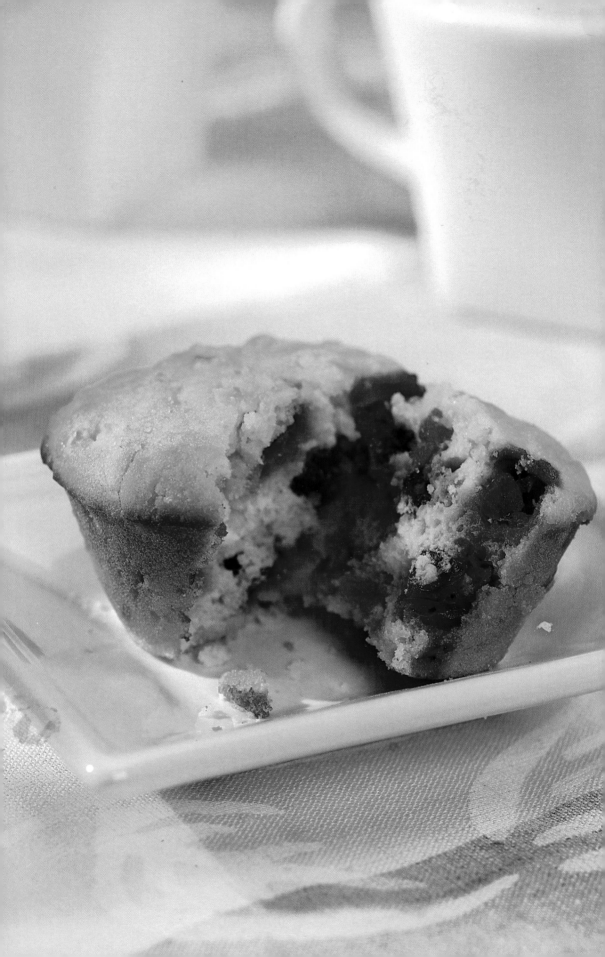

Cranberry Orange Muffins

MAKES 12 MUFFINS

Each muffin is dotted with bright red cranberries and flavored with a hint of orange. The cake-like texture of this not-too-sweet muffin is perfect to serve warm for breakfast.

TIP
Leave cranberries in the freezer until just before using. This prevents them from "bleeding" into the bread. Sprinkle a little granulated sugar on top, just before baking, to help them brown.

VARIATIONS
For a sweeter muffin, replace fresh or frozen cranberries with dried.

∽

You can also substitute fresh or frozen blueberries for the cranberries.

Preheat oven to 350°F (180°C)
Muffin tin, lightly greased

1½ cups	rice flour	375 mL
⅓ cup	cornstarch	75 mL
⅓ cup	tapioca starch	75 mL
1½ tsp	xanthan gum	7 mL
1 tbsp	GF baking powder	15 mL
¾ tsp	salt	4 mL
⅔ cup	cranberry juice	150 mL
⅓ cup	water	75 mL
⅔ cup	orange marmalade	150 mL
1 tsp	cider vinegar	5 mL
¼ cup	vegetable oil	50 mL
2	eggs	2
1 cup	cranberries, fresh or frozen	250 mL

1. In a large bowl, stir together rice flour, cornstarch, tapioca starch, xanthan gum, baking powder and salt. Set aside.

2. In a separate bowl, using an electric mixer, beat cranberry juice, water, marmalade, vinegar, oil and eggs until combined.

3. Pour marmalade mixture over dry ingredients and stir just until combined. Gently fold in cranberries. Spoon into each cup of prepared muffin tin. Let stand for 30 minutes.

4. Bake in preheated oven for 25 to 30 minutes or until firm to the touch and tops are golden. Remove from the pan immediately and let cool completely on a rack.

Cranberry Orange Muffins (page 65)

Mock Date Bran Muffins

MAKES 12 MUFFINS

Dark, moist and full of fruit! Serve these with a crisp apple and a wedge of five-year-old Cheddar.

TIPS

These muffins remain moist longer than most. Carry them when you travel.

∽

If you purchase chopped dates, check the packaging for hidden gluten in the coating.

VARIATIONS

Substitute raisins or dried figs for the dates.

∽

Spoon batter into a lightly greased 9-by 5-inch (2 L) loaf pan and bake for 70 to 80 minutes or until a cake tester inserted in the center comes out clean.

Preheat oven to 350°F (180°C)
Muffin tin, lightly greased

1 cup	sorghum flour	250 mL
½ cup	whole bean flour	125 mL
⅓ cup	tapioca starch	75 mL
⅓ cup	rice bran	75 mL
2 tsp	xanthan gum	10 mL
1 tsp	GF baking powder	5 mL
½ tsp	baking soda	2 mL
¼ tsp	salt	1 mL
1 cup	chopped dates	250 mL
1½ cups	buttermilk	375 mL
¼ cup	vegetable oil	50 mL
2	eggs	2
¼ cup	liquid honey	50 mL
2 tbsp	fancy molasses	25 mL

1. In a large bowl, stir together sorghum flour, whole bean flour, tapioca starch, rice bran, xanthan gum, baking powder, baking soda, salt and dates. Set aside.

2. In a separate bowl, using an electric mixer, beat buttermilk, oil and eggs until combined. Add honey and molasses while mixing.

3. Pour buttermilk mixture over dry ingredients and stir just until combined. Spoon into each cup of prepared muffin tin. Let stand for 30 minutes.

4. Bake in preheated oven for 25 to 30 minutes or until firm to the touch. Remove from the pan immediately and let cool completely on a rack.

Orange Pecan Streusel Muffins

MAKES 12 MUFFINS

> *What an attractive, tasty treat! The golden crunchy streusel topping contrasts beautifully with the bright orange flecks of this muffin.*

TIPS

Remove the muffins carefully from the pan or the topping will shake off.

∾

If muffins stick to the pan, let stand for 2 to 3 minutes, then try again. To provide space for the topping, fill each muffin cup only three-quarters full.

∾

If pecan flour is not readily available in your area, make your own (see Nut Flour, page 180).

VARIATION

Substitute sunflower seeds for the pecans.

Preheat oven to 350°F (180°C)
Muffin tin, lightly greased

TOPPING

¼ cup	packed brown sugar	50 mL
2 tbsp	pecan flour	25 mL
½ tsp	ground cinnamon	2 mL
1 tbsp	melted butter	15 mL

MUFFIN

1 cup	rice flour	250 mL
⅓ cup	pecan flour	75 mL
¼ cup	tapioca starch	50 mL
¼ cup	potato starch	50 mL
½ cup	granulated sugar	125 mL
1½ tsp	xanthan gum	7 mL
2 tsp	GF baking powder	10 mL
¼ tsp	baking soda	1 mL
½ tsp	salt	2 mL
2 tbsp	orange zest	25 mL
½ cup	chopped pecans	125 mL
¾ cup	orange juice	175 mL
¼ cup	vegetable oil	50 mL
2	eggs	2

1. In a small bowl, combine brown sugar, pecan flour and cinnamon. Add melted butter and mix until crumbly. Set aside streusel topping.

2. In a large bowl, stir together rice flour, pecan flour, tapioca starch, potato starch, sugar, xanthan gum, baking powder, baking soda, salt, orange zest and pecans. Set aside.

3. In a separate bowl, using an electric mixer or whisk, beat orange juice, oil and eggs until combined. Pour over dry ingredients and stir just until combined. Spoon into prepared muffin tin. Sprinkle streusel topping over batter. Let stand for 30 minutes.

4. Bake in preheated oven for 25 to 30 minutes or until firm to the touch. Remove from the pan immediately and let cool completely on a rack.

Zucchini Carrot Muffins

Here's an exceptionally attractive muffin — confetti dots of bright orange carrot contrast with the brilliant green of zucchini.

TIPS

For moister muffins, choose young carrots and zucchini fresh from the garden.

If muffins stick to the pan, let stand 2 to 3 minutes, then try again.

We found these muffins took a little longer to bake than others in this book.

VARIATION

Add ¾ cup (175 mL) chopped walnuts, pecans or sunflower seeds with the dry ingredients.

Preheat oven to 350°F (180°C)
Muffin tin, lightly greased

1²⁄₃ cups	sorghum flour	400 mL
⅓ cup	tapioca starch	75 mL
⅓ cup	potato starch	75 mL
⅓ cup	granulated sugar	75 mL
1½ tsp	xanthan gum	7 mL
2 tsp	GF baking powder	10 mL
½ tsp	salt	2 mL
¾ tsp	ground cinnamon	4 mL
¼ tsp	ground allspice	1 mL
¼ tsp	ground nutmeg	1 mL
1 cup	milk	250 mL
1 tsp	cider vinegar	5 mL
¼ cup	vegetable oil	50 mL
2	eggs	2
1 cup	unpeeled, grated zucchini	250 mL
1 cup	grated carrots	250 mL

1. In a large bowl, stir together sorghum flour, tapioca starch, potato starch, sugar, xanthan gum, baking powder, salt, cinnamon, allspice and nutmeg. Set aside.

2. In a separate bowl, using an electric mixer or whisk, beat milk, vinegar, oil and eggs until combined.

3. Pour milk mixture over dry ingredients and stir just until combined. Fold in zucchini and carrots. Spoon into each cup of prepared muffin tin. Let stand for 30 minutes.

4. Bake in preheated oven for 35 to 40 minutes or until firm to the touch. Remove from the pan immediately and let cool completely on a rack.

Blueberry Buckwheat Loaf

If you enjoy blueberry buckwheat pancakes, you'll love the intriguing flavor of this speckled dark loaf.

TIPS

If using frozen blueberries, leave them in the freezer until ready to use. This helps to prevent them from "bleeding" into the loaf.

∽

Stir the dry ingredients thoroughly before liquids are added — the rice flour and starches are so finely textured, they clump very easily.

VARIATIONS

Substitute chopped prunes, figs or plums for the blueberries.

∽

If your diet does not permit buckwheat flour, you can replace it with soy or sorghum flour.

Preheat oven to 350°F (180°C)
9-by 5-inch (2 L) loaf pan, lightly greased

³⁄₄ cup	brown rice flour	175 mL
¼ cup	buckwheat flour	50 mL
¼ cup	potato starch	50 mL
¼ cup	tapioca starch	50 mL
1½ tsp	xanthan gum	7 mL
2 tsp	GF baking powder	10 mL
1 tsp	baking soda	5 mL
½ tsp	salt	2 mL
1¼ cups	buttermilk	300 mL
1 tsp	cider vinegar	5 mL
¼ cup	vegetable oil	50 mL
2	eggs	2
½ cup	liquid honey	125 mL
1 cup	blueberries, fresh or frozen (see Tip, left)	250 mL

1. In a large bowl, stir together brown rice flour, buckwheat flour, potato starch, tapioca starch, xanthan gum, baking powder, baking soda and salt. Set aside.

2. In a separate bowl, using an electric mixer, beat buttermilk, vinegar, oil and eggs until combined. Add honey while mixing.

3. Pour buttermilk mixture over dry ingredients and stir just until combined. Gently fold in blueberries. Spoon into prepared pan. Let stand for 30 minutes.

4. Bake in preheated oven for 70 to 80 minutes or until a cake tester inserted in the center comes out clean. Let cool in the pan on a rack for 10 minutes. Remove from the pan and let cool completely on a rack.

Country Harvest Loaf

MAKES 1 LOAF

This is one of our favorite flavor combinations. The seeds add an interesting texture and crunch to the loaf.

TIPS

Flaxseed needs to be slightly cracked or ground to be easily digested. Slightly crack the flaxseed in a blender, coffee mill or food processor.

∾

To prevent seeds from becoming rancid, store in an airtight container in the refrigerator.

VARIATIONS

Vary the combination of seeds. Try poppy, pumpkin or whatever kind of seeds you prefer.

∾

Prepare a dozen muffins instead of a loaf. Follow the method of any muffin recipe in this chapter. Bake for 20 to 30 minutes or until firm to the touch.

Preheat oven to 350°F (180°C)
9-by 5-inch (2 L) loaf pan, lightly greased

1¼ cups	rice flour	300 mL
⅓ cup	cornstarch	75 mL
⅓ cup	tapioca starch	75 mL
1½ tsp	xanthan gum	7 mL
1 tbsp	GF baking powder	15 mL
¾ tsp	salt	4 mL
⅓ cup	cracked flaxseed (see Tip, left)	75 mL
⅓ cup	sunflower seeds	75 mL
2 tbsp	sesame seeds	25 mL
1 cup	milk	250 mL
1 tsp	cider vinegar	5 mL
⅓ cup	vegetable oil	75 mL
2	eggs	2
½ cup	liquid honey	125 mL

1. In a large bowl, stir together rice flour, cornstarch, tapioca starch, xanthan gum, baking powder, salt, flaxseed, sunflower seeds and sesame seeds. Set aside.

2. In a separate bowl, using an electric mixer, beat milk, vinegar, oil and eggs until combined. Add honey while mixing.

3. Pour milk mixture over dry ingredients and stir just until combined. Spoon into prepared pan. Let stand for 30 minutes.

4. Bake in preheated oven for 65 to 75 minutes or until a cake tester inserted in the center comes out clean. Let cool in the pan on a rack for 10 minutes. Remove from the pan and let cool completely on a rack.

Glazed Lemon Coconut Loaf

MAKES 1 LOAF

Brown rice flour gives this loaf — a delightfully sweet tea bread — a warm creamy color. Bake ahead and freeze it, so it's ready the next time a friend drops in.

TIP

Use either desiccated or shredded coconut in this recipe. If using a sweetened coconut, decrease the sugar by 1 or 2 tbsp (15 or 25 mL).

VARIATION

Orange zest and orange juice can replace the lemon for a slightly sweeter and more mild-flavored loaf.

Preheat oven to 350°F (180°C)
9-by 5-inch (2 L) loaf pan, lightly greased

1 cup	brown rice flour	250 mL
1/3 cup	potato starch	75 mL
1/4 cup	tapioca starch	50 mL
1 cup	granulated sugar	250 mL
1 1/2 tsp	xanthan gum	7 mL
1 tbsp	GF baking powder	15 mL
1/4 tsp	salt	1 mL
2 tbsp	lemon zest	25 mL
3/4 cup	unsweetened coconut (see Tip, left)	175 mL
3/4 cup	milk	175 mL
1/4 cup	vegetable oil	50 mL
2	eggs	2
1/4 cup	freshly squeezed lemon juice	50 mL

LEMON GLAZE

1 cup	GF sifted confectioner's (icing) sugar	250 mL
1/4 cup	freshly squeezed lemon juice	50 mL

1. In a large bowl, stir together brown rice flour, potato starch, tapioca starch, sugar, xanthan gum, baking powder, salt, zest and coconut. Set aside.

2. In a separate bowl, using an electric mixer or whisk, beat milk, oil and eggs until combined. Add lemon juice while mixing. Pour milk mixture over dry ingredients and stir just until combined. Spoon into prepared pan. Let stand for 30 minutes.

3. Bake in preheated oven for 55 to 65 minutes or until a cake tester inserted in the center comes out clean.

4. Meanwhile, prepare Lemon Glaze. In a small bowl, stir together confectioner's sugar and lemon juice. With a wooden skewer, poke several holes through the hot loaf as soon as it is removed from the oven. Spoon the glaze over the hot loaf. Let the loaf cool in the pan on a rack for 30 minutes. Remove from the pan and let cool completely on a rack.

Peppered Zucchini Loaf

MAKES 1 LOAF

Confetti-like speckles of zucchini and bell pepper add to the moistness of this flavorful loaf. It's perfect for sandwiches or to serve along with a salad or stew.

TIPS

Use red, orange or yellow bell peppers or a combination of colors.

∾

To increase the fiber content, do not peel the zucchini.

VARIATIONS

For a little extra heat, substitute some chili or jalapeño pepper for a small amount of the bell pepper.

∾

If you prefer a dozen muffins, follow the method of any muffin recipe in this chapter. Bake for 30 to 40 minutes or until firm to the touch.

Preheat oven to 350°F (180°C)
9-by 5-inch (2 L) loaf pan, lightly greased

1 cup	rice flour	250 mL
2/3 cup	tapioca starch	150 mL
1/3 cup	cornstarch	75 mL
1/4 cup	granulated sugar	50 mL
1 1/2 tsp	xanthan gum	7 mL
2 tsp	GF baking powder	10 mL
1/2 tsp	salt	2 mL
1/4 tsp	freshly ground black pepper	1 mL
3/4 cup	buttermilk	175 mL
1 tsp	cider vinegar	5 mL
1/4 cup	vegetable oil	50 mL
2	eggs	2
1 cup	unpeeled, shredded zucchini	250 mL
1/2 cup	finely chopped bell peppers (see Tip, left)	125 mL

1. In a large bowl, stir together rice flour, tapioca starch, cornstarch, sugar, xanthan gum, baking powder, salt and black pepper. Set aside.
2. In a separate bowl, using an electric mixer or whisk, beat buttermilk, vinegar, oil and eggs until combined.
3. Pour buttermilk mixture over dry ingredients and stir just until combined. Fold in zucchini and bell peppers. Spoon into prepared pan. Let stand for 30 minutes.
4. Bake in preheated oven for 70 to 80 minutes or until a cake tester inserted in the center comes out clean. Let cool in the pan on a rack for 10 minutes. Remove from the pan and let cool completely on a rack.

Pumpkin Seed Loaf

MAKES 1 LOAF

> *Don't be put off by the long list of ingredients — nothing could be faster or easier than this comfort food.*

TIPS

For a nuttier flavor, toast the pumpkin and sunflower seeds (see Techniques Glossary, page 180, for instructions).

∾

Pumpkin pie spice may contain gluten fillers.

VARIATION

Use your favorite combination of sweet spices instead of ginger, nutmeg and cloves.

Preheat oven to 350°F (180°C)
9-by 5-inch (2 L) loaf pan, lightly greased

¾ cup	sorghum flour	175 mL
¾ cup	whole bean flour	175 mL
¼ cup	cornstarch	50 mL
⅔ cup	packed brown sugar	150 mL
1½ tsp	xanthan gum	7 mL
2 tsp	GF baking powder	10 mL
2 tsp	baking soda	10 mL
½ tsp	salt	2 mL
1 tsp	ground ginger	5 mL
½ tsp	ground nutmeg	2 mL
¼ tsp	ground cloves	1 mL
⅓ cup	pumpkin seeds	75 mL
⅓ cup	sunflower seeds	75 mL
1 cup	canned pumpkin purée (not pie filling)	250 mL
1 tsp	cider vinegar	5 mL
⅓ cup	vegetable oil	75 mL
2	eggs	2

1. In a large bowl, stir together sorghum flour, whole bean flour, cornstarch, brown sugar, xanthan gum, baking powder, baking soda, salt, ginger, nutmeg, cloves, pumpkin seeds and sunflower seeds. Set aside.

2. In a separate bowl, using an electric mixer or whisk, beat pumpkin purée, vinegar, oil and eggs until combined.

3. Pour pumpkin mixture over dry ingredients and stir just until combined. Spoon into prepared pan. Let stand for 30 minutes.

4. Bake in preheated oven for 70 to 80 minutes or until a cake tester inserted in the center comes out clean. Let cool in the pan on a rack for 10 minutes. Remove from the pan and let cool completely on a rack.

Swedish Limpa Loaf

MAKES 1 LOAF

> *The traditional Scandinavian flavor combination of anise, caraway and fennel seeds gives this orange-scented loaf a unique flavor.*

TIP

For a smoother texture, use a food mill or a coffee mill to grind the seeds.

VARIATION

Vary the combination of seeds. Try poppy or sesame. For a milder-flavored version of the loaf, omit the seeds.

Preheat oven to 350°F (180°C)
9-by 5-inch (2 L) loaf pan, lightly greased

²/₃ cup	whole bean flour	150 mL
¹/₂ cup	sorghum flour	125 mL
¹/₂ cup	potato starch	125 mL
¹/₂ cup	tapioca starch	125 mL
¹/₂ cup	packed brown sugar	125 mL
2 tsp	xanthan gum	10 mL
2 tsp	GF baking powder	10 mL
³/₄ tsp	salt	4 mL
1 tbsp	orange zest	15 mL
2 tsp	anise seeds	10 mL
2 tsp	caraway seeds	10 mL
2 tsp	fennel seeds	10 mL
1¹/₄ cups	milk	300 mL
1 tsp	cider vinegar	5 mL
¹/₄ cup	vegetable oil	50 mL
2	eggs	2

1. In a large bowl, stir together whole bean flour, sorghum flour, potato starch, tapioca starch, brown sugar, xanthan gum, baking powder, salt, orange zest, anise seeds, caraway seeds and fennel seeds. Set aside.

2. In a separate bowl, using an electric mixer or whisk, beat milk, vinegar, oil and eggs until combined. Pour mixture over dry ingredients and stir just until combined. Spoon into prepared pan. Let stand for 30 minutes.

3. Bake in preheated oven for 70 to 80 minutes or until a cake tester inserted in the center comes out clean. Let cool in the pan on a rack for 10 minutes. Remove from the pan and let cool completely on a rack.

Fresh Tomato Basil Drop Biscuits

MAKES 14 BISCUITS

These biscuits are packed with the flavor of late summer — juicy, sweet tomatoes and the pungent fragrance of fresh basil.

TIP

In season, use garden-fresh beefsteak tomatoes. Use an Italian plum or Roma tomato at other times of the year. Leave tomatoes in fairly large pieces.

VARIATION

Substitute an equal amount of plain yogurt for the gluten-free sour cream.

Preheat oven to 425°F (220°C)
Baking sheet, lightly greased

¾ cup	rice flour	175 mL
¼ cup	tapioca starch	50 mL
¼ cup	potato starch	50 mL
2 tbsp	granulated sugar	25 mL
1 tsp	xanthan gum	5 mL
1 tbsp	GF baking powder	15 mL
¼ tsp	salt	2 mL
¼ cup	snipped fresh basil	50 mL
¼ cup	snipped fresh chives	50 mL
¼ cup	snipped fresh parsley	50 mL
¼ cup	shortening	50 mL
¾ cup	chopped fresh tomatoes (see Tip, left)	175 mL
½ cup	GF sour cream	125 mL

1. In a large bowl, stir together rice flour, tapioca starch, potato starch, sugar, xanthan gum, baking powder, salt, basil, chives and parsley.

2. Using a pastry blender or two knives, cut in shortening until mixture resembles coarse crumbs. Fold in tomatoes. Add sour cream all at once, stirring with a fork to make a soft, sticky dough. Drop by heaping tablespoonfuls (15 mL) onto prepared pan. Let stand for 30 minutes.

3. Bake in preheated oven for 12 to 15 minutes or until tops are golden. Remove to a cooling rack immediately. Serve warm.

Rosemary Scones Topped with Caramelized Vidalia Onions

MAKES 6 WEDGES

> *What a lunch treat! Just cut into wedges and serve hot from the oven with a crisp salad.*

TIPS

For long, thin onion slices, cut the onion in half lengthwise before slicing.

∾

For instructions on caramelizing onions, see Techniques Glossary, page 180.

Preheat oven to 425°F (220°C)
8-inch (20 cm) round baking pan, lightly greased

TOPPING

1 tbsp	butter	15 mL
2 cups	sliced Vidalia onions (see Tip, left)	500 mL
1½ tsp	packed brown sugar	7 mL
2 tbsp	snipped fresh rosemary leaves	25 mL

BASE

¾ cup	brown rice flour	175 mL
¼ cup	arrowroot starch	50 mL
¼ cup	potato starch	50 mL
1½ tsp	granulated sugar	7 mL
1 tsp	xanthan gum	5 mL
2 tsp	GF baking powder	10 mL
½ tsp	baking soda	2 mL
½ tsp	salt	2 mL
2 tbsp	snipped fresh rosemary leaves	25 mL
¼ cup	cold butter, cut into 1-inch (2.5 cm) cubes	50 mL
1	egg	1
⅔ cup	buttermilk	150 mL

VARIATIONS

Substitute fresh oregano or basil for the rosemary.

❧

When Vidalia onions are out of season, try Spanish onions instead.

❧

Spoon batter into 4 lightly greased English muffin rings placed on a baking sheet, three-quarters full. Do not press the dough down, spread with topping and bake for 12 to 15 minutes or until tops are golden.

1. *Topping:* In a large frying pan, melt butter over medium heat. Add onions, stirring frequently, until tender and a deep golden brown, about 20 minutes. Remove from heat. Stir in brown sugar and rosemary. Set aside to cool.

2. *Base:* In a large bowl, stir together brown rice flour, arrowroot starch, potato starch, sugar, xanthan gum, baking powder, baking soda, salt and rosemary.

3. Using a pastry blender or two knives, cut in butter until mixture resembles coarse crumbs.

4. In a small bowl, whisk together egg and buttermilk. Add to flour mixture all at once, stirring with a fork to make a soft, sticky dough. Spoon into prepared pan, spread evenly, leaving top rough. Let stand for 30 minutes. Spread with topping.

5. Bake in preheated oven for 20 to 25 minutes or until top is golden. Remove to a cooling rack immediately. Cut into 6 wedges. Serve warm.

Lemon Yogurt Scones

MAKES 5
LARGE BISCUITS
OR 8 DROP BISCUITS

Tangy with yogurt and lemon, these biscuits, served warm from the oven, quickly become a favorite!

TIP
Cold butter cuts more easily into dry ingredients than soft butter and it produces flakier biscuits. For easier handling, first cut the butter into 1-inch (2.5 cm) cubes.

VARIATION
For a delicious shortcake biscuit, add an extra 1 tbsp (15 mL) granulated sugar to the dry ingredients. Top with sliced fresh strawberries, peaches or raspberries in season. Serve with whipped cream.

Preheat oven to 425°F (220°C)
English muffin rings placed on a baking sheet and lightly greased (see Equipment Glossary, page 171)

1 cup	white rice flour	250 mL
1/3 cup	arrowroot starch	75 mL
1/3 cup	potato starch	75 mL
2 tbsp	granulated sugar	25 mL
1 tsp	xanthan gum	5 mL
1 tbsp	GF baking powder	15 mL
1/2 tsp	baking soda	2 mL
1 tbsp	lemon zest	15 mL
1/2 tsp	salt	2 mL
1/3 cup	cold butter, cut into 1-inch (2.5 cm) cubes (see Tip, left)	75 mL
1 cup	plain yogurt	250 mL

1. In a large bowl, stir together rice flour, arrowroot starch, potato starch, sugar, xanthan gum, baking powder, baking soda, lemon zest and salt.

2. Using a pastry blender or two knives, cut in butter until mixture resembles coarse crumbs. Add yogurt all at once, stirring with a fork to make a soft, sticky dough.

3. Spoon into rings, three-quarters full. If desired, smooth tops with wet fingers or a small spatula but do not press the dough down or drop by heaping tablespoonfuls (15 mL) onto greased baking sheet. Let stand for 30 minutes.

4. Bake in preheated oven for 12 to 15 minutes or until top is golden. Remove to a cooling rack immediately. Remove from rings and serve warm.

Yeast Breads from Your Bread Machine

Our favorite appliance! Delicious homemade breads with none of the work! These same recipes are also found in Mixer-Method Yeast Breads on page 95, for those of you who don't own a bread machine.

~ Bread Machine ~ Yeast Baking

- The recipes in this chapter are developed for 1.5 lb (750 g) and 2 lb (1 kg) bread machines. Choose a machine with a vigorous kneading action. We find the vertical machines consistently produce better loaves than those baking horizontal loaves.

- Choose a machine that has a Rapid 2-Hour Basic Cycle, a Dough and a Bake Cycle or a machine with a Programmable Cycle.

- Set the Programmable Cycle to have a short knead of 2 minutes (the machine stirs slowly, allowing for the addition of the dry ingredients). Then set a knead of 20 minutes, then a rise of 70 minutes and a 50-minute bake cycle at 350°F (180°C). When prompted, set all the others to 0, eliminating the extra cycles.

- Allow the eggs to mix with the liquid ingredients in the bread machine for 1 to 2 minutes before adding the dry ingredients.

- Carefully scrape the corners, sides and bottom of the baking pan and the kneading blade while adding the dry ingredients. Watch that the rubber spatula does not get caught under the rotating kneading blade. Continue scraping until the mixture is smooth and lump-free.

- The consistency of the dough is closer to a cake batter than traditional yeast bread dough. You should see the motion of the kneading blade turning and the dough should be shiny, not dull. The mixing mark of the kneading blade remains on the top of the dough.

- For machines without the Programmable Cycle, remove the kneading blade just after the long knead stops. This prevents over-kneading, which may result in a collapsed loaf. Because gluten-free products are sticky, rinse the rubber spatula and your hand with cold water before removing the blade. Smooth the top of the loaf but resist handling the dough too much.

- When using the Dough and then Bake Cycle, notice whether your machine knocks down the dough just before the Dough Cycle ends. If it does, stop the cycle 5 minutes before the end. Set a separate kitchen timer to remind you. The dough is risen and ready to bake. Just press the Bake Cycle. There's no need to handle the dough at all.

- Wrap loaves while still warm and let cool completely. Slice bread with an electric knife or bread knife with a serrated blade and wrap each slice individually, then place slices in a second resealable bag. Freeze them for up to 3 weeks. Remove 1 or 2 slices as required.

Banana Seed Bread

MAKES 1 LOAF

The combination of sorghum and bean flour really enhances the banana flavor of this loaf. Serve it for dessert or with a slice of old Cheddar for lunch.

TIP

Use raw, unroasted, unsalted sunflower seeds. For a nuttier flavor, toast the sunflower seeds (see Techniques Glossary, page 180, for instructions).

VARIATION

Pumpkin seeds or chopped pecans can replace the sunflower seeds.

1 cup	whole bean flour	250 mL
1 cup	sorghum flour	250 mL
¼ cup	tapioca starch	50 mL
¼ cup	packed brown sugar	50 mL
2 ½ tsp	xanthan gum	12 mL
1 tbsp	bread machine or instant yeast	15 mL
1 ¼ tsp	salt	6 mL
½ cup	sunflower seeds (see Tip, left)	125 mL
¾ cup	water	175 mL
1 cup	mashed banana	250 mL
1 tsp	cider vinegar	5 mL
¼ cup	vegetable oil	50 mL
2	eggs	2

1. In a large bowl or plastic bag, combine whole bean flour, sorghum flour, tapioca starch, brown sugar, xanthan gum, yeast, salt and sunflower seeds. Mix well and set aside.

2. Pour water, banana, vinegar and oil into the bread machine baking pan. Add eggs.

3. Select the Rapid 2-Hour Basic Cycle. Allow the liquids to mix until combined. Gradually add the dry ingredients as the bread machine is mixing. Scrape with a rubber spatula while adding the dry ingredients. Try to incorporate all the dry ingredients within 1 to 2 minutes. When mixing and kneading are complete, leaving the bread pan in the bread machine, remove the kneading blade. Allow the bread machine to complete the cycle.

Brown Bread

MAKES 1 LOAF

The perfect sandwich bread! Just add shaved roast beef, a leaf of romaine and a hint of mustard. It carries well for a tasty lunch.

TIP
Slice this or any bread with an electric knife for thin, even sandwich slices.

VARIATIONS
For a mild-flavored bread, substitute 2 tbsp (25 mL) packed brown sugar for the molasses.

∿

The rice bran can be replaced by an equal amount of brown or white rice flour.

1 1/2 cups	brown rice flour	375 mL
1/2 cup	sorghum flour	125 mL
1/2 cup	cornstarch	125 mL
1/2 cup	rice bran	125 mL
1 tbsp	xanthan gum	15 mL
1 tbsp	bread machine or instant yeast	15 mL
1 1/4 tsp	salt	6 mL
1 cup	water	250 mL
1 tsp	cider vinegar	5 mL
2 tbsp	vegetable oil	25 mL
2 tbsp	liquid honey	25 mL
2 tbsp	fancy molasses	25 mL
3	eggs	3

1. In a large bowl or plastic bag, combine brown rice flour, sorghum flour, cornstarch, rice bran, xanthan gum, yeast and salt. Mix well and set aside.

2. Pour water, vinegar, oil, honey and molasses into the bread machine baking pan. Add eggs.

3. Select the Rapid 2-Hour Basic Cycle. Allow the liquids to mix until combined. Gradually add the dry ingredients as the bread machine is mixing. Scrape with a rubber spatula while adding the dry ingredients. Try to incorporate all the dry ingredients within 1 to 2 minutes. When the mixing and kneading are complete, leaving the bread pan in the bread machine, remove the kneading blade. Allow the bread machine to complete the cycle.

Buckwheat Walnut

This is the bread for those who love to combine strong, robust flavors — buckwheat, whole bean flour and cardamom.

TIP

Make sure buckwheat is on your list of allowable foods before you try this recipe.

VARIATIONS

Substitute brown rice flour for the buckwheat flour.

❧

Substitute fresh, dried or frozen blueberries for the walnuts. Fold the fruit in just at the end of the kneading cycle.

❧

Substitute an equal amount of nutmeg for the cardamom.

1 1/4 cups	whole bean flour	300 mL
1/2 cup	buckwheat flour	125 mL
1/2 cup	potato starch	125 mL
1/4 cup	tapioca starch	50 mL
1/3 cup	packed brown sugar	75 mL
1 tbsp	xanthan gum	15 mL
1 tbsp	bread machine or instant yeast	15 mL
1 1/4 tsp	salt	6 mL
1 tsp	ground cardamom	5 mL
1 cup	chopped walnuts	250 mL
1 3/4 cups	water	425 mL
1 tsp	cider vinegar	5 mL
1/4 cup	vegetable oil	50 mL
2	eggs	2

1. In a large bowl or plastic bag, combine whole bean flour, buckwheat flour, potato starch, tapioca starch, brown sugar, xanthan gum, yeast, salt, cardamom and walnuts. Mix well and set aside.

2. Pour water, vinegar and oil into the bread machine baking pan. Add eggs.

3. Select the Rapid 2-Hour Basic Cycle. Allow the liquids to mix until combined. Gradually add the dry ingredients as the bread machine is mixing. Scrape with a rubber spatula while adding the dry ingredients. Try to incorporate all the dry ingredients within 1 to 2 minutes. When the mixing and kneading are complete, leaving the bread pan in the bread machine, remove the kneading blade. Allow the bread machine to complete the cycle.

Cheese Onion Loaf

MAKES 1 LOAF

This is a perfect accompaniment to homemade chili or beef stew. It slices well and stays moist for a second day.

TIPS

Do not substitute fresh onion for the dried flakes. The extra moisture results in a weak-flavored shorter loaf.

∿

For the amount of cheese to purchase, see the weight/volume equivalents in the Ingredient Glossary, page 173.

VARIATION

Monterey Jack, Parmesan or Swiss cheese could be substituted for the Cheddar. Try a combination but do not exceed the total volume in the recipe or the loaf will be short and heavy.

1$\frac{2}{3}$ cups	rice flour	400 mL
$\frac{2}{3}$ cup	sorghum flour	150 mL
$\frac{1}{3}$ cup	arrowroot starch	75 mL
$\frac{1}{4}$ cup	nonfat dry milk or skim milk powder	50 mL
2 tbsp	granulated sugar	25 mL
1 tbsp	xanthan gum	15 mL
1 tbsp	bread machine or instant yeast	15 mL
1$\frac{1}{4}$ tsp	salt	6 mL
1 cup	shredded old Cheddar cheese	250 mL
2 tbsp	dried onion flakes (see Tip, left)	25 mL
$\frac{1}{4}$ tsp	dry mustard	1 mL
1 cup	water	250 mL
2 tsp	cider vinegar	10 mL
2	eggs	2
2	egg whites	2

1. In a large bowl or plastic bag, combine rice flour, sorghum flour, arrowroot starch, milk powder, sugar, xanthan gum, yeast, salt, cheese, onion flakes and mustard. Mix well and set aside.

2. Pour water and vinegar into bread machine baking pan. Add eggs and egg whites.

3. Select the Rapid 2-Hour Basic Cycle. Allow the liquids to mix until combined. Gradually add the dry ingredients as the bread machine is mixing. Scrape with a rubber spatula while adding the dry ingredients. Try to incorporate all the dry ingredients within 1 to 2 minutes. When the mixing and kneading are complete, leaving the bread pan in the bread machine, remove the kneading blade. Allow the bread machine to complete the cycle.

Cornbread

Tiny bits of moist kernel corn dot this warm-colored yellow loaf.

TIP
Drain the canned corn before measuring. If using frozen corn, thaw and drain before measuring.

VARIATION
Add $1/4$ cup (50 mL) grated Parmesan cheese or $1/4$ cup (50 mL) finely chopped red and green bell peppers.

1 $1/4$ cups	rice flour	300 mL
1 cup	cornmeal	250 mL
$1/2$ cup	potato starch	125 mL
$1/4$ cup	tapioca starch	50 mL
3 tbsp	granulated sugar	45 mL
1 tbsp	xanthan gum	15 mL
1 tbsp	bread machine or instant yeast	15 mL
1 $1/4$ tsp	salt	6 mL
1 $1/4$ cups	water	300 mL
1 tsp	cider vinegar	5 mL
$1/4$ cup	vegetable oil	50 mL
$1/2$ cup	well-drained whole corn kernels (see Tip, left)	125 mL
4	eggs	4

1. In a large bowl or plastic bag, combine rice flour, cornmeal, potato starch, tapioca starch, sugar, xanthan gum, yeast and salt. Mix well and set aside.

2. Pour water, vinegar, oil and corn into bread machine baking pan. Add eggs.

3. Select the Rapid 2-Hour Basic Cycle. Allow the liquids to mix until combined. Gradually add the dry ingredients as the bread machine is mixing. Scrape with a rubber spatula while adding the dry ingredients. Try to incorporate all the dry ingredients within 1 to 2 minutes. When the mixing and kneading are complete, leaving the bread pan in the bread machine, remove the kneading blade. Allow the bread machine to complete the cycle.

Cranberry Wild Rice Loaf

MAKES 1 LOAF

This attractive loaf is sure to bring compliments from guests. The nutty taste with a hint of orange makes this a perfect accompaniment for duck or turkey.

VARIATION
Substitute raspberry or orange-flavored dried cranberries.

1½ cups	brown rice flour	375 mL
⅔ cup	tapioca starch	150 mL
⅓ cup	potato starch	75 mL
¼ cup	granulated sugar	50 mL
2½ tsp	xanthan gum	12 mL
2 tsp	bread machine or instant yeast	10 mL
1½ tsp	salt	7 mL
2 tsp	orange zest	10 mL
¾ tsp	celery seeds	4 mL
⅛ tsp	freshly ground black pepper	0.5 mL
1 cup	cooked wild rice (see Techniques Glossary, page 180)	250 mL
¾ cup	dried cranberries	175 mL
1 cup	water	250 mL
¼ cup	frozen orange juice concentrate, thawed	50 mL
¼ cup	vegetable oil	50 mL
2	eggs	2
2	egg whites	2

1. In a large bowl or plastic bag, combine brown rice flour, tapioca starch, potato starch, sugar, xanthan gum, yeast, salt, zest, celery seeds, black pepper, wild rice and cranberries. Mix well and set aside.

2. Pour water, orange juice concentrate and oil into the bread machine baking pan. Add eggs and egg whites.

3. Select the Rapid 2-Hour Basic Cycle. Allow the liquids to mix until combined. Gradually add the dry ingredients as the bread machine is mixing. Scrape with a rubber spatula while adding the dry ingredients. Try to incorporate all the dry ingredients within 1 to 2 minutes. When the mixing and kneading are complete, leaving the bread pan in the bread machine, remove the kneading blade. Allow the bread machine to complete the cycle.

Sun-Dried Tomato Rice Loaf

MAKES 1 LOAF

For those who prefer savory loaves to sweet, try this variation of the Cranberry Wild Rice Loaf suggested by Larry, a member of our focus group.

TIP

Select dry, not oil-packed, sun-dried tomatoes.

VARIATION

Substitute ¼ cup (50 mL) frozen orange juice concentrate, thawed, for the same amount of water.

1½ cups	brown rice flour	375 mL
⅔ cup	tapioca starch	150 mL
⅓ cup	potato starch	75 mL
¼ cup	granulated sugar	50 mL
2½ tsp	xanthan gum	12 mL
2 tsp	bread machine or instant yeast	10 mL
½ tsp	salt	2 mL
¾ tsp	celery seeds	4 mL
¼ tsp	freshly ground black pepper	1 mL
1 cup	cooked wild rice (see Techniques Glossary, page 180)	250 mL
⅔ cup	sun-dried tomatoes (see Tip, left)	150 mL
1¼ cups	water	300 mL
¼ cup	vegetable oil	50 mL
2	eggs	2
2	egg whites	2

1. In a large bowl or plastic bag, combine brown rice flour, tapioca starch, potato starch, sugar, xanthan gum, yeast, salt, celery seeds, pepper, wild rice and sun-dried tomatoes. Mix well and set aside.

2. Pour water and oil into the bread machine baking pan. Add eggs and egg whites.

3. Select the Rapid Two-Hour Basic Cycle. Allow the liquids to mix until combined. Gradually add the dry ingredients as the bread machine is mixing, scraping with a rubber spatula. Try to incorporate all the dry ingredients within 1 to 2 minutes. When the mixing and kneading are complete, leaving the bread pan in the bread machine, remove the kneading blade. Allow the bread machine to complete the cycle.

Cottage Cheese Dill Loaf

MAKES 1 LOAF

Try this twist on a traditional white bread to serve along with salmon or your favorite seafood entrée.

TIP

Any type of cottage cheese — large or small curd, high or low fat — works well in this recipe.

VARIATION

Omit the dill. Try rosemary, marjoram or savory.

2 cups	rice flour	500 mL
2/3 cup	potato starch	150 mL
1/3 cup	tapioca starch	75 mL
2 1/2 tsp	xanthan gum	12 mL
2 tsp	bread machine or instant yeast	10 mL
1 1/2 tsp	salt	7 mL
1 tbsp	snipped fresh dill	15 mL
1 cup	water	250 mL
1 tsp	cider vinegar	5 mL
1/2 cup	low-fat cottage cheese (see Tip, left)	125 mL
1/4 cup	vegetable oil	50 mL
1/4 cup	liquid honey	50 mL
4	eggs	4

1. In a large bowl or plastic bag, combine rice flour, potato starch, tapioca starch, xanthan gum, yeast, salt and dill. Mix well and set aside.

2. Pour water, vinegar, cottage cheese, oil and honey into bread machine baking pan. Add eggs.

3. Select the Rapid 2-Hour Basic Cycle. Allow the liquids to mix until combined. Gradually add the dry ingredients as the bread machine is mixing. Scrape with a rubber spatula while adding the dry ingredients. Try to incorporate all the dry ingredients within 1 to 2 minutes. When the mixing and kneading are complete, leaving the bread pan in the bread machine, remove the kneading blade. Allow the bread machine to complete the cycle.

Flaxseed with Banana Bread

MAKES 1 LOAF

> *Toasting a slice brings out the banana flavor. No need to butter this bread.*

VARIATION

Pancake syrup (light or regular) or packed brown sugar can be substituted for the pure maple syrup.

1½ cups	brown rice flour	375 mL
⅔ cup	potato starch	150 mL
⅓ cup	tapioca starch	75 mL
1 tbsp	xanthan gum	15 mL
2 tsp	bread machine or instant yeast	10 mL
1½ tsp	salt	7 mL
⅓ cup	cracked flaxseed (see Techniques Glossary, page 179)	75 mL
¾ cup	water	175 mL
1 cup	mashed banana	250 mL
2 tsp	cider vinegar	10 mL
¼ cup	vegetable oil	50 mL
¼ cup	pure maple syrup	50 mL
2	eggs	2
2	egg whites	2

1. In a large bowl or plastic bag, combine brown rice flour, potato starch, tapioca starch, xanthan gum, yeast, salt and flaxseed. Mix well and set aside.

2. Pour water, banana, vinegar, oil and maple syrup into the bread machine baking pan. Add eggs and egg whites.

3. Select the Rapid 2-Hour Basic Cycle. Allow liquids to mix until combined. Gradually add the dry ingredients as the bread machine is mixing. Scrape with a rubber spatula while adding the dry ingredients. Try to incorporate all the dry ingredients within 1 to 2 minutes. When the mixing and kneading are complete, leaving the bread pan in the bread machine, remove the kneading blade. Allow the bread machine to complete the cycle.

Lemon Poppy Loaf

MAKES 1 LOAF

A perennial favorite flavor combination — poppy seeds and lemon.

TIPS

Use a zester to make long thin strips of lemon zest. Be sure to remove only the colored outer skin, avoiding the bitter white pith beneath.

∾

Freshly squeezed lemon juice enhances the flavor. Roll the lemon on the counter or between your hands to loosen the juice.

∾

Keep a lemon in the freezer. Zest while frozen, then juice after warming in the microwave.

VARIATION

Substitute double the amount of orange zest for lemon and use orange juice instead of lemon juice.

1 1/2 cups	rice flour	375 mL
2/3 cup	potato starch	150 mL
1/3 cup	arrowroot starch	75 mL
1/3 cup	granulated sugar	75 mL
1 tbsp	xanthan gum	15 mL
1 tbsp	bread machine or instant yeast	15 mL
1 1/4 tsp	salt	6 mL
2 tbsp	lemon zest (see Tips, left)	25 mL
1/3 cup	poppy seeds	75 mL
1 1/4 cups	water	300 mL
1/4 cup	freshly squeezed lemon juice (see Tips, left)	50 mL
1/4 cup	vegetable oil	50 mL
2	eggs	2
2	egg whites	2

1. In a large bowl or plastic bag, combine rice flour, potato starch, arrowroot starch, sugar, xanthan gum, yeast, salt, zest and poppy seeds. Mix well and set aside.

2. Pour water, lemon juice and oil into the bread machine baking pan. Add eggs and egg whites.

3. Select the Rapid 2-Hour Basic Cycle. Allow the liquids to mix until combined. Gradually add the dry ingredients as the bread machine is mixing. Scrape with a rubber spatula while adding the dry ingredients. Try to incorporate all the dry ingredients within 1 to 2 minutes. When the mixing and kneading are complete, leaving the bread pan in the bread machine, remove the kneading blade. Allow the bread machine to complete the cycle.

Nutmeg Loaf

MAKES 1 LOAF

Flecks of brown nutmeg stand out against the white background in this tangy-sweet loaf. The aroma will have you slicing it hot.

TIP

For the best flavor, use freshly grated whole nutmeg. Use approximately half as much fresh grated as ground.

VARIATIONS

If you cannot tolerate quinoa or it is unavailable, increase the rice flour by $1/3$ cup (75 mL).

∾

Vanilla yogurt or gluten-free sour cream can replace the plain yogurt. Read the label carefully because some contain wheat starch.

1 $1/4$ cups	brown rice flour	300 mL
$1/2$ cup	arrowroot starch	125 mL
$1/4$ cup	quinoa flour (see Variations, left)	50 mL
$1/4$ cup	tapioca starch	50 mL
$1/3$ cup	granulated sugar	75 mL
1 tbsp	xanthan gum	15 mL
1 tbsp	bread machine or instant yeast	15 mL
1 $1/4$ tsp	salt	6 mL
1 $1/2$ tsp	ground nutmeg (see Tip, left)	7 mL
$1/3$ cup	water	75 mL
$1/2$ cup	plain yogurt	125 mL
$1/4$ cup	vegetable oil	50 mL
2	eggs	2

1. In a large bowl or plastic bag, combine rice flour, arrowroot starch, quinoa flour, tapioca starch, sugar, xanthan gum, yeast, salt and nutmeg. Mix well and set aside.

2. Pour water, yogurt and oil into the bread machine baking pan. Add eggs.

3. Select the Rapid 2-Hour Basic Cycle. Allow the liquids to mix until combined. Gradually add the dry ingredients as the bread machine is mixing. Scrape with a rubber spatula while adding the dry ingredients. Try to incorporate all the dry ingredients within 1 to 2 minutes. When the mixing and kneading are complete, leaving the bread pan in the bread machine, remove the kneading blade. Allow the bread machine to complete the cycle.

Pumpernickel Loaf

TIP

Remember to thoroughly mix the dry ingredients before adding to the liquids because they are powder-fine and could clump together.

VARIATIONS

If yellow pea flour is unavailable, use chickpea or garbanzo bean flour. This recipe can either be made from any variety of bean flour or half pea and half bean flour.

∾

For a milder flavor, omit the coffee and unsweetened cocoa powder.

1 cup	whole bean flour	250 mL
1 cup	yellow pea flour (see Variations, left)	250 mL
⅔ cup	potato starch	150 mL
⅓ cup	tapioca starch	75 mL
3 tbsp	packed brown sugar	45 mL
2½ tsp	xanthan gum	12 mL
1 tbsp	bread machine or instant yeast	15 mL
1½ tsp	salt	7 mL
1 tbsp	instant coffee granules	15 mL
1 tbsp	unsweetened cocoa powder	15 mL
½ tsp	ground ginger	2 mL
1½ cups	water	375 mL
3 tbsp	fancy molasses	45 mL
1 tsp	cider vinegar	5 mL
2 tbsp	vegetable oil	25 mL
3	eggs	3

1. In a large bowl or plastic bag, combine whole bean flour, yellow pea flour, potato starch, tapioca starch, brown sugar, xanthan gum, yeast, salt, coffee granules, cocoa and ginger. Mix well and set aside.

2. Pour water, molasses, vinegar and oil into the bread machine baking pan. Add eggs.

3. Select the Rapid 2-Hour Basic Cycle. Allow the liquids to mix until combined. Gradually add the dry ingredients as the bread machine is mixing. Scrape with a rubber spatula while adding the dry ingredients. Try to incorporate all the dry ingredients within 1 to 2 minutes. When the mixing and kneading are complete, leaving the bread pan in the bread machine, remove the kneading blade. Allow the bread machine to complete the cycle.

Tomato Rosemary Bread

MAKES 1 LOAF

A smaller loaf than some, this is just the size to accompany an Italian dinner!

TIPS

The tomato vegetable juice should be at room temperature. If using cold from the refrigerator, heat it on High in the microwave for 1 minute.

∽

When substituting fresh herbs for the dried, triple the amount.

∽

Use dry (not oil-packed) sun-dried tomatoes.

VARIATION

Vary the herb — select oregano, basil or thyme.

1 cup	sorghum flour	250 mL
½ cup	whole bean flour	125 mL
½ cup	cornstarch	125 mL
¼ cup	granulated sugar	50 mL
1 tbsp	xanthan gum	15 mL
1 tbsp	bread machine or instant yeast	15 mL
½ tsp	salt	2 mL
2 tsp	dried rosemary	10 mL
½ cup	snipped sun-dried tomatoes	125 mL
1¼ cups	tomato vegetable juice (see Tips, left)	300 mL
¼ cup	vegetable oil	50 mL
2	eggs	2

1. In a large bowl or plastic bag, combine sorghum flour, whole bean flour, cornstarch, sugar, xanthan gum, yeast, salt, rosemary and tomatoes. Mix well and set aside.

2. Pour juice and oil into the bread machine baking pan. Add eggs.

3. Select the Rapid 2-Hour Basic Cycle. Allow the liquids to mix until combined. Gradually add the dry ingredients as the bread machine is mixing. Scrape with a rubber spatula while adding the dry ingredients. Try to incorporate all the dry ingredients within 1 to 2 minutes. When the mixing and kneading are complete, leaving the bread pan in the bread machine, remove the kneading blade. Allow the bread machine to complete the cycle.

White Bread

We know you'll enjoy this moist all-purpose yeast bread, whether for sandwiches or to accompany your favorite salad.

TIPS

Remember to thoroughly mix the dry ingredients before adding to the liquids because they are powder-fine and could clump together.

∾

Use any leftovers to make bread crumbs (see Techniques Glossary, page 178).

VARIATION

Add 1¼ cups (300 mL) milk instead of the water and nonfat dry milk or skim milk powder.

2 cups	rice flour	500 mL
⅔ cup	potato starch	150 mL
⅓ cup	tapioca starch	75 mL
¼ cup	nonfat dry milk or skim milk powder	50 mL
¼ cup	granulated sugar	50 mL
2½ tsp	xanthan gum	12 mL
2¼ tsp	bread machine or instant yeast	11 mL
1½ tsp	salt	7 mL
1¼ cups	water	300 mL
1 tsp	cider vinegar	5 mL
¼ cup	vegetable oil	50 mL
2	eggs	2
2	egg whites	2

1. In a large bowl or plastic bag, combine rice flour, potato starch, tapioca starch, milk powder, sugar, xanthan gum, yeast and salt. Mix well and set aside.

2. Pour water, vinegar and oil into the bread machine baking pan. Add eggs and egg whites.

3. Select the Rapid 2-Hour Basic Cycle. Allow the liquids to mix until combined. Gradually add the dry ingredients as the bread machine is mixing. Scrape with a rubber spatula while adding the dry ingredients. Try to incorporate all the dry ingredients within 1 to 2 minutes. When the mixing and kneading are complete, leaving the bread pan in the bread machine, remove the kneading blade. Allow the bread machine to complete the cycle.

Mixer-Method Yeast Breads

These same recipes are also found in Yeast Breads from Your Bread Machine on page 79. They have the same wonderful flavors and are the perfect size for a loaf baked in the oven.

~ Mixer-Method ~ Yeast Baking

- Select a heavy-duty stand mixer to make gluten-free yeast breads. A lighter hand-held mixer may not be powerful enough to handle the thicker doughs.

- Use the paddle attachment. The dough is not thick enough to knead with the dough hook and yet too thick for the wire whip.

- If flours contain lumps, sift before measuring. Combine all the dry ingredients in a plastic bag or a large bowl before adding to the mixer bowl. Gluten-free flours and starches have a fine, powder-like consistency and lump easily unless mixed with other dry ingredients.

- Mix the eggs with the liquid ingredients on low speed for 1 to 2 minutes or until blended before adding the dry ingredients.

- Add the dry ingredients slowly as the machine is mixing. Stop the mixer and scrape the sides and bottom of the bowl and the blade with a rubber spatula.

- With the mixer set to medium speed, beat the dough for 4 minutes. Set a kitchen timer. You will be surprised how long 4 minutes actually seems as you wait.

- Scrape the dough into a lightly greased baking pan. It should fill the pan about two-thirds full. If too full, the loaf does not bake with a rounded top, similar to a wheat loaf, but overflows the sides, leaving a slightly flat top and mushroomed sides.

- Set aside to rise in a warm, draft-free place until the dough reaches the top of the pan. We leave them uncovered because the dough sticks if it touches any kind of cover. Do not let it over-rise — the loaf will mushroom slightly and collapse during baking, if over-risen.

- Test whether the bread is done with an instant-read metal stem thermometer inserted at least 2 inches (5 cm) into the loaf. The thermometer should register 190°F (90°C). A long wooden skewer, inserted in the center of the loaf, should come out clean. Tap on the bottom of the loaf and if the sound is hollow, the bread is baked.

- Remove from the pan to a wire rack immediately to prevent a soggy loaf. Cool completely on a wire rack.

- Slice and wrap while still warm in airtight individual sandwich bags, then place these in a larger freezer bag. Label and date, then freeze up to 6 weeks. For thin, even slices, use an electric knife or one with a serrated blade.

Banana Seed Bread

MAKES 1 LOAF

The combination of sorghum and bean flour really enhances the banana flavor of this loaf. Serve it for dessert or with a slice of old Cheddar for lunch.

TIP

Use raw, unroasted, unsalted sunflower seeds. For a nuttier flavor, toast the sunflower seeds (see Techniques Glossary, page 180, for instructions).

VARIATION

Pumpkin seeds or chopped pecans can replace the sunflower seeds.

9-by 5-inch (2 L) loaf pan, lightly greased

¾ cup	whole bean flour	175 mL
¾ cup	sorghum flour	175 mL
¼ cup	tapioca starch	50 mL
¼ cup	packed brown sugar	50 mL
2 tsp	xanthan gum	10 mL
1 tbsp	bread machine or instant yeast	15 mL
1 tsp	salt	5 mL
½ cup	sunflower seeds (see Tip, left)	125 mL
½ cup	water	125 mL
¾ cup	mashed banana	175 mL
1 tsp	cider vinegar	5 mL
3 tbsp	vegetable oil	45 mL
2	eggs	2

1. In a large bowl or plastic bag, combine whole bean flour, sorghum flour, tapioca starch, brown sugar, xanthan gum, yeast, salt and sunflower seeds. Mix well and set aside.

2. In a separate bowl, using a heavy-duty electric mixer with paddle attachment, combine water, banana, vinegar, oil and eggs until well blended.

3. With the mixer on lowest speed, slowly add the dry ingredients to the banana mixture until combined. With a rubber spatula, scrape the bottom and sides of the bowl. With the mixer on medium speed, beat for 4 minutes.

4. Spoon into prepared pan. Let rise, uncovered, in a warm, draft-free place for 60 to 75 minutes or until the dough has risen to the top of the pan. Meanwhile, preheat oven to 350°F (180°C). Tent with foil and bake for 20 to 25 minutes. Remove foil and continue baking for 15 to 20 minutes more or until the loaf sounds hollow when tapped on the bottom.

Brown Bread

MAKES 1 LOAF

The perfect sandwich bread! Just add shaved roast beef, a leaf of romaine and a hint of mustard. It carries well for a tasty lunch.

TIP
Slice this or any bread with an electric knife for thin, even sandwich slices.

VARIATIONS
For a mild-flavored bread, substitute 2 tbsp (25 mL) packed brown sugar for the molasses.

∽

The rice bran can be replaced by an equal amount of brown or white rice flour.

9-by 5-inch (2 L) loaf pan, lightly greased

1¼ cups	brown rice flour	300 mL
½ cup	sorghum flour	125 mL
½ cup	cornstarch	125 mL
½ cup	rice bran	125 mL
1 tbsp	xanthan gum	15 mL
1 tbsp	bread machine or instant yeast	15 mL
1¼ tsp	salt	6 mL
1 cup	water	250 mL
1 tsp	cider vinegar	5 mL
2 tbsp	vegetable oil	25 mL
2 tbsp	liquid honey	25 mL
2 tbsp	fancy molasses	25 mL
3	eggs	3

1. In a large bowl or plastic bag, combine brown rice flour, sorghum flour, cornstarch, rice bran, xanthan gum, yeast and salt. Mix well and set aside.

2. In a separate bowl, using a heavy-duty electric mixer with paddle attachment, combine water, vinegar, oil, honey, molasses and eggs until well blended.

3. With the mixer on lowest speed, slowly add the dry ingredients to the honey mixture until combined. With a rubber spatula, scrape the bottom and sides of the bowl. With the mixer on medium speed, beat for 4 minutes.

4. Spoon into prepared pan. Let rise, uncovered, in a warm, draft-free place for 60 to 75 minutes or until the dough has risen to the top of the pan. Meanwhile, preheat oven to 350°F (180°C). Bake for 35 to 45 minutes or until the loaf sounds hollow when tapped on the bottom.

Buckwheat Walnut

This is the bread for those who love to combine strong, robust flavors — buckwheat, whole bean flour and cardamom.

TIP

Make sure buckwheat is on your list of allowable foods before you try this recipe.

VARIATIONS

Substitute brown rice flour for the buckwheat flour.

∽

Substitute fresh, dried or frozen blueberries for the walnuts. Fold the fruit in just before spooning into pan.

∽

Substitute an equal amount of nutmeg for the cardamom.

9-by 5-inch (2 L) loaf pan, lightly greased

1 cup	whole bean flour	250 mL
1/3 cup	buckwheat flour	75 mL
1/2 cup	potato starch	125 mL
1/4 cup	tapioca starch	50 mL
1/4 cup	packed brown sugar	50 mL
2 tsp	xanthan gum	10 mL
1 tbsp	bread machine or instant yeast	15 mL
1 tsp	salt	5 mL
3/4 tsp	ground cardamom	4 mL
3/4 cup	chopped walnuts	175 mL
1 1/4 cups	water	300 mL
1 tsp	cider vinegar	5 mL
3 tbsp	vegetable oil	45 mL
2	eggs	2

1. In a large bowl or plastic bag, combine whole bean flour, buckwheat flour, potato starch, tapioca starch, brown sugar, xanthan gum, yeast, salt, cardamom and walnuts. Mix well and set aside.

2. In a separate bowl, using a heavy-duty electric mixer with paddle attachment, combine water, vinegar, oil and eggs until well blended.

3. With the mixer on lowest speed, slowly add the dry ingredients until combined. With a rubber spatula, scrape the bottom and sides of the bowl. With the mixer on medium speed, beat for 4 minutes.

4. Spoon into prepared pan. Let rise, uncovered, in a warm, draft-free place for 60 to 75 minutes or until the dough has risen to the top of the pan. Meanwhile, preheat oven to 350°F (180°C). Bake for 35 to 45 minutes or until the loaf sounds hollow when tapped on the bottom.

Cheese Onion Loaf

MAKES 1 LOAF

This is a perfect accompaniment to homemade chili or beef stew. It slices well and stays moist for a second day.

TIPS

Do not substitute fresh onion for the dried flakes. The extra moisture results in a weak-flavored shorter loaf.

∽

For the amount of cheese to purchase, see the weight/volume equivalents in the Ingredient Glossary, page 173.

VARIATION

Monterey Jack, Parmesan or Swiss cheese could be substituted for the Cheddar. Try a combination but do not exceed the total volume in the recipe, or the loaf will be short and heavy.

9-by 5-inch (2 L) loaf pan, lightly greased

1½ cups	rice flour	375 mL
½ cup	sorghum flour	125 mL
⅓ cup	arrowroot starch	75 mL
¼ cup	nonfat dry milk or skim milk powder	50 mL
2 tbsp	granulated sugar	25 mL
2½ tsp	xanthan gum	12 mL
2 tsp	bread machine or instant yeast	10 mL
1¼ tsp	salt	6 mL
¾ cup	shredded old Cheddar cheese	175 mL
2 tbsp	dried onion flakes (see Tips, left)	25 mL
¼ tsp	dry mustard	1 mL
1¼ cups	water	300 mL
2 tsp	cider vinegar	10 mL
2	eggs	2
2	egg whites	2

1. In a large bowl or plastic bag, combine rice flour, sorghum flour, arrowroot starch, milk powder, sugar, xanthan gum, yeast, salt, cheese, onion flakes and mustard. Mix well and set aside.

2. In a separate bowl, using a heavy-duty electric mixer with paddle attachment, combine water, vinegar, eggs and egg whites until well blended.

3. With the mixer on lowest speed, slowly add the dry ingredients until combined. With a rubber spatula, scrape the bottom and sides of the bowl. With the mixer on medium speed, beat for 4 minutes.

4. Spoon into prepared pan. Let rise, uncovered, in a warm, draft-free place for 60 to 75 minutes or until the dough has risen to the top of the pan. Meanwhile, preheat oven to 350°F (180°C). Bake for 35 to 45 minutes or until the loaf sounds hollow when tapped on the bottom.

Cornbread

Tiny bits of moist kernel corn dot this warm-colored yellow loaf.

TIP

Drain the canned corn before measuring. If using frozen corn, thaw and drain before measuring.

VARIATION

Add ¼ cup (50 mL) grated Parmesan cheese or ¼ cup (50 mL) finely chopped red and green bell peppers.

9-by 5-inch (2 L) loaf pan, lightly greased

1 cup	rice flour	250 mL
¾ cup	cornmeal	175 mL
⅓ cup	potato starch	75 mL
¼ cup	tapioca starch	50 mL
2 tbsp	granulated sugar	25 mL
1 tbsp	xanthan gum	15 mL
1 tbsp	bread machine or instant yeast	15 mL
1 tsp	salt	5 mL
½ cup	well-drained whole corn kernels (see Tip, left)	125 mL
1 cup	water	250 mL
1 tsp	cider vinegar	5 mL
¼ cup	vegetable oil	50 mL
2	eggs	2

1. In a large bowl or plastic bag, combine rice flour, cornmeal, potato starch, tapioca starch, sugar, xanthan gum, yeast, salt and corn. Mix well and set aside.

2. In a separate bowl, using a heavy-duty electric mixer with paddle attachment, combine water, vinegar, oil and eggs until well blended.

3. With the mixer on lowest speed, slowly add the dry ingredients until combined. With a rubber spatula, scrape the bottom and sides of the bowl. With the mixer on medium speed, beat for 4 minutes.

4. Spoon into prepared pan. Let rise, uncovered, in a warm, draft-free place for 60 to 75 minutes or until the dough has risen to the top of the pan. Meanwhile, preheat oven to 350°F (180°C). Bake for 35 to 45 minutes or until the loaf sounds hollow when tapped on the bottom.

Cranberry Wild Rice Loaf

This attractive loaf is sure to bring compliments from guests. The nutty taste with a hint of orange makes this a perfect accompaniment for duck or turkey.

VARIATION

Substitute raspberry or orange-flavored dried cranberries.

9-by 5-inch (2 L) loaf pan, lightly greased

1¼ cups	brown rice flour	300 mL
½ cup	tapioca starch	125 mL
¼ cup	potato starch	50 mL
3 tbsp	granulated sugar	45 mL
2½ tsp	xanthan gum	12 mL
2 tsp	bread machine or instant yeast	10 mL
1½ tsp	salt	7 mL
2 tsp	orange zest	10 mL
¾ tsp	celery seeds	4 mL
⅛ tsp	fleshly ground black pepper	0.5 mL
¾ cup	cooked wild rice (see Techniques Glossary, page 180)	175 mL
½ cup	dried cranberries	125 mL
¾ cup	water	175 mL
¼ cup	frozen orange juice concentrate, thawed	50 mL
¼ cup	vegetable oil	50 mL
2	eggs	2
1	egg white	1

1. In a large bowl or plastic bag, combine brown rice flour, tapioca starch, potato starch, sugar, xanthan gum, yeast, salt, zest, celery seeds, pepper, wild rice and cranberries. Mix well and set aside.

2. In a separate bowl, using a heavy-duty electric mixer with paddle attachment, combine water, orange juice concentrate, oil, eggs and egg white until well blended.

3. With the mixer on lowest speed, slowly add the dry ingredients until combined. With a rubber spatula, scrape the bottom and sides of the bowl. With the mixer on medium speed, beat for 4 minutes.

4. Spoon into prepared pan. Let rise, uncovered, in a warm, draft-free place for 60 to 75 minutes or until the dough has risen to the top of the pan. Meanwhile, preheat oven to 350°F (180°C). Bake for 35 to 45 minutes or until the loaf sounds hollow when tapped on the bottom.

Sun-Dried Tomato Rice Loaf

MAKES 1 LOAF

> For those who prefer savory loaves to sweet, try this variation of the Cranberry Wild Rice Loaf suggested by Larry, a member of our focus group.

TIP

Select dry, not oil-packed, sun-dried tomatoes.

VARIATION

Substitute ¼ cup (50 mL) frozen orange juice concentrate, thawed, for the same amount of water.

9-by 5-inch (2 L) loaf pan, lightly greased

1¼ cups	brown rice flour	300 mL
½ cup	tapioca starch	125 mL
¼ cup	potato starch	50 mL
3 tbsp	granulated sugar	45 mL
2½ tsp	xanthan gum	12 mL
2 tsp	bread machine or instant yeast	10 mL
½ tsp	salt	2 mL
¾ tsp	celery seeds	4 mL
⅛ tsp	freshly ground black pepper	0.5 mL
¾ cup	cooked wild rice (see Techniques Glossary, page 180)	175 mL
⅓ cup	sun-dried tomatoes (see Tip, left)	75 mL
1 cup	water	250 mL
¼ cup	vegetable oil	50 mL
2	eggs	2
1	egg white	1

1. In a large bowl or plastic bag, combine brown rice flour, tapioca starch, potato starch, sugar, xanthan gum, yeast, salt, celery seeds, pepper, wild rice and sun-dried tomatoes. Mix well and set aside.

2. In a separate bowl, using a heavy-duty electric mixer with paddle attachment, combine water, oil, eggs and egg white until well combined.

3. With the mixer on lowest speed, slowly add the dry ingredients until combined. With a rubber spatula, scrape the bottom and sides of the bowl. With the mixer on medium speed, beat for 4 minutes.

4. Spoon into prepared pan. Let rise, uncovered, in a warm, draft-free place for 60 to 75 minutes or until the dough has risen to the top of the pan. Meanwhile, preheat oven to 350°F (180°C). Bake for 35 to 45 minutes or until the loaf sounds hollow when tapped on the bottom.

Cottage Cheese Dill Loaf

MAKES 1 LOAF

Try this twist on a traditional white bread to serve along with salmon or your favorite seafood entrée.

TIP

Any type of cottage cheese — large or small curd, high or low fat — works well in this recipe.

VARIATION

Omit the dill. Try rosemary, marjoram or savory.

9-by 5-inch (2 L) loaf pan, lightly greased

1½ cups	rice flour	375 mL
½ cup	potato starch	125 mL
¼ cup	tapioca starch	50 mL
2¼ tsp	xanthan gum	11 mL
2 tsp	bread machine or instant yeast	10 mL
1½ tsp	salt	7 mL
1 tbsp	snipped fresh dill	15 mL
¾ cup	water	175 mL
1 tsp	cider vinegar	5 mL
½ cup	low-fat cottage cheese (see Tip, left)	125 mL
2 tbsp	vegetable oil	25 mL
3 tbsp	liquid honey	45 mL
2	eggs	2
2	egg whites	2

1. In a large bowl or plastic bag, combine rice flour, potato starch, tapioca starch, xanthan gum, yeast, salt and dill. Mix well and set aside.

2. In a separate bowl, using a heavy-duty electric mixer with paddle attachment, combine water, vinegar, cottage cheese, oil, honey, eggs and egg whites until well blended.

3. With the mixer on lowest speed, slowly add the dry ingredients until combined. With a rubber spatula, scrape the bottom and sides of the bowl. With the mixer on medium speed, beat for 4 minutes.

4. Spoon into prepared pan. Let rise, uncovered, in a warm, draft-free place for 60 to 75 minutes or until the dough has risen to the top of the pan. Meanwhile, preheat oven to 350°F (180°C). Bake for 35 to 45 minutes or until the loaf sounds hollow when tapped on the bottom.

Flaxseed with Banana Bread

MAKES 1 LOAF

Toasting a slice brings out the banana flavor. No need to butter this bread.

VARIATION
Liquid honey or packed brown sugar can be substituted for the maple syrup.

9-by 5-inch (2 L) loaf pan, lightly greased

1⅓ cups	brown rice flour	325 mL
⅓ cup	potato starch	75 mL
¼ cup	tapioca starch	50 mL
1 tbsp	xanthan gum	15 mL
2 tsp	bread machine or instant yeast	10 mL
1¼ tsp	salt	6 mL
¼ cup	cracked flaxseed (see Techniques Glossary, page 179)	50 mL
⅔ cup	water	150 mL
¾ cup	mashed banana	175 mL
1 tsp	cider vinegar	5 mL
¼ cup	vegetable oil	50 mL
3 tbsp	pure maple syrup	45 mL
2	eggs	2

1. In a large bowl or plastic bag, combine brown rice flour, potato starch, tapioca starch, xanthan gum, yeast, salt and flaxseed. Mix well and set aside.

2. In a separate bowl, using a heavy-duty electric mixer with paddle attachment, combine water, banana, vinegar, oil, maple syrup and eggs until well blended.

3. With the mixer on lowest speed, slowly add the dry ingredients until combined. With a rubber spatula, scrape the bottom and sides of the bowl. With the mixer on medium speed, beat for 4 minutes.

4. Spoon into prepared pan. Let rise, uncovered, in a warm, draft-free place for 60 to 75 minutes or until the dough has risen to the top of the pan. Meanwhile, preheat oven to 350°F (180°C). Bake for 35 to 45 minutes or until the loaf sounds hollow when tapped on the bottom.

Lemon Poppy Loaf

A perennial favorite flavor combination — poppy seeds and lemon.

TIPS

Use a zester to make long thin strips of lemon zest. Be sure to remove only the colored outer skin, avoiding the bitter white pith beneath.

∾

Freshly squeezed lemon juice enhances the flavor. Roll the lemon on the counter or between your hands to loosen the juice.

∾

Keep a lemon in the freezer. Zest while frozen, then juice after warming in the microwave.

VARIATION

Substitute double the amount of orange zest for lemon and use orange juice instead of lemon juice.

9-by 5-inch (2 L) loaf pan, lightly greased

1¼ cups	rice flour	300 mL
½ cup	potato starch	125 mL
¼ cup	arrowroot starch	50 mL
¼ cup	granulated sugar	50 mL
1 tbsp	xanthan gum	15 mL
1 tbsp	bread machine or instant yeast	15 mL
1 tsp	salt	5 mL
2 tbsp	lemon zest (see Tips, left)	25 mL
¼ cup	poppy seeds	50 mL
1 cup	water	250 mL
¼ cup	freshly squeezed lemon juice (see Tips, left)	50 mL
3 tbsp	vegetable oil	45 mL
2	eggs	2
1	egg white	1

1. In a large bowl or plastic bag, combine rice flour, potato starch, arrowroot starch, sugar, xanthan gum, yeast, salt, zest and poppy seeds. Mix well and set aside.

2. In a separate bowl, using a heavy-duty electric mixer with paddle attachment, combine water, lemon juice, oil, eggs and egg white until well blended.

3. With the mixer on lowest speed, slowly add the dry ingredients until combined. With a rubber spatula, scrape the bottom and sides of the bowl. With the mixer on medium speed, beat for 4 minutes.

4. Spoon into prepared pan. Let rise, uncovered, in a warm, draft-free place for 60 to 75 minutes or until the dough has risen to the top of the pan. Meanwhile, preheat oven to 350°F (180°C). Bake for 35 to 45 minutes or until the loaf sounds hollow when tapped on the bottom.

Nutmeg Loaf

MAKES 1 LOAF

9-by 5-inch (2 L) loaf pan, lightly greased

TIP

For the best flavor, use freshly grated whole nutmeg. Use approximately half as much freshly grated as ground.

VARIATIONS

If you cannot tolerate quinoa or it is unavailable, increase the rice flour by ⅓ cup (75 mL).

❧

Vanilla yogurt or gluten-free sour cream can replace the plain yogurt. Read the label carefully because some contain wheat starch.

1¼ cups	brown rice flour	300 mL
⅓ cup	arrowroot starch	75 mL
⅓ cup	quinoa flour (see Variations, left)	75 mL
¼ cup	tapioca starch	50 mL
2 tbsp	granulated sugar	25 mL
1 tbsp	xanthan gum	15 mL
1 tbsp	bread machine or instant yeast	15 mL
1¼ tsp	salt	6 mL
1¼ tsp	ground nutmeg (see Tips, left)	6 mL
⅔ cup	water	150 mL
⅔ cup	plain yogurt	150 mL
¼ cup	vegetable oil	50 mL
2	eggs	2

1. In a large bowl or plastic bag, combine rice flour, arrowroot starch, quinoa flour, tapioca starch, sugar, xanthan gum, yeast, salt and nutmeg. Mix well and set aside.

2. In a separate bowl, using a heavy-duty electric mixer with paddle attachment, combine water, yogurt, oil and eggs until well blended.

3. With the mixer on lowest speed, slowly add the dry ingredients until combined. With a rubber spatula, scrape the bottom and sides of the bowl. With the mixer on medium speed, beat for 4 minutes.

4. Spoon into prepared pan. Let rise, uncovered, in a warm, draft-free place for 60 to 75 minutes or until the dough has risen to the top of the pan. Meanwhile, preheat oven to 350°F (180°C). Bake for 35 to 45 minutes or until the loaf sounds hollow when tapped on the bottom.

Pumpernickel Loaf

MAKES 1 LOAF

TIP

Remember to
thoroughly mix the
dry ingredients before
adding to the liquids
because they are
powder-fine and could
clump together.

VARIATIONS

If yellow pea flour
is unavailable, use
chickpea or garbanzo
bean flour. This recipe
can either be made from
any variety of bean flour
or half pea and half
bean flour.

∾

For a milder flavor,
omit the coffee
and unsweetened
cocoa powder.

9-by 5-inch (2 L) loaf pan, lightly greased

¾ cup	whole bean flour	175 mL
¾ cup	yellow pea flour (see Variations, left)	175 mL
½ cup	potato starch	125 mL
¼ cup	tapioca starch	50 mL
2 tbsp	packed brown sugar	25 mL
2 tsp	xanthan gum	10 mL
1 tbsp	bread machine or instant yeast	15 mL
1¼ tsp	salt	6 mL
2 tsp	instant coffee granules	10 mL
2 tsp	unsweetened cocoa powder	10 mL
½ tsp	ground ginger	2 mL
1¼ cups	water	300 mL
2 tbsp	fancy molasses	25 mL
1 tsp	cider vinegar	5 mL
2 tbsp	vegetable oil	25 mL
2	eggs	2

1. In a large bowl or plastic bag, combine whole bean flour, yellow pea flour, potato starch, tapioca starch, brown sugar, xanthan gum, yeast, salt, coffee granules, cocoa and ginger. Mix well and set aside.

2. In a separate bowl, using a heavy-duty electric mixer with paddle attachment, combine water, molasses, vinegar, oil and eggs until well blended.

3. With the mixer on lowest speed, slowly add the dry ingredients until combined. With a rubber spatula, scrape the bottom and sides of the bowl. With the mixer on medium speed, beat for 4 minutes.

4. Spoon into prepared pan. Let rise, uncovered, in a warm, draft-free place for 60 to 75 minutes or until the dough has risen to the top of the pan. Meanwhile, preheat oven to 350°F (180°C). Bake for 35 to 45 minutes or until the loaf sounds hollow when tapped on the bottom.

Tomato Rosemary Bread

MAKES 1 LOAF

9-by 5-inch (2 L) loaf pan, lightly greased

> *A smaller loaf than some, this is just the size to accompany an Italian dinner!*

TIPS

The tomato vegetable juice should be at room temperature. If using cold from the refrigerator, heat it on High in the microwave for 1 minute.

∿

When substituting fresh herbs for the dried, triple the amount.

∿

Use dry (not oil-packed) sun-dried tomatoes.

VARIATION

Vary the herb — select oregano, basil or thyme.

1 cup	sorghum flour	250 mL
½ cup	whole bean flour	125 mL
⅓ cup	cornstarch	75 mL
3 tbsp	granulated sugar	45 mL
1 tbsp	xanthan gum	15 mL
1 tbsp	bread machine or instant yeast	15 mL
½ tsp	salt	2 mL
1½ tsp	dried rosemary	7 mL
⅓ cup	snipped sun-dried tomatoes	75 mL
1¼ cups	tomato vegetable juice (see Tips, left)	300 mL
¼ cup	vegetable oil	50 mL
2	eggs	2

1. In a large bowl or plastic bag, combine sorghum flour, whole bean flour, cornstarch, sugar, xanthan gum, yeast, salt, rosemary and tomatoes. Mix well and set aside.

2. In a separate bowl, using a heavy-duty electric mixer with paddle attachment, combine juice, oil and eggs until well blended.

3. With the mixer on lowest speed, slowly add the dry ingredients until combined. With a rubber spatula, scrape the bottom and sides of the bowl. With the mixer on medium speed, beat for 4 minutes.

4. Spoon into prepared pan. Let rise, uncovered, in a warm, draft-free place for 60 to 75 minutes or until the dough has risen to the top of the pan. Meanwhile, preheat oven to 350°F (180°C). Bake for 35 to 45 minutes or until the loaf sounds hollow when tapped on the bottom.

White Bread

We know you'll enjoy this moist all-purpose yeast bread, whether for sandwiches or to accompany your favorite salad.

TIPS

Remember to thoroughly mix the dry ingredients before adding to the liquids because they are powder-fine and could clump together.

∽

Use any leftovers to make bread crumbs (see Techniques Glossary, page 178).

9-by 5-inch (2 L) loaf pan, lightly greased

1¾ cups	rice flour	425 mL
½ cup	potato starch	125 mL
¼ cup	tapioca starch	50 mL
¼ cup	nonfat dry milk or skim milk powder	50 mL
2 tbsp	granulated sugar	25 mL
2½ tsp	xanthan gum	12 mL
2 tsp	bread machine or instant yeast	10 mL
1¼ tsp	salt	6 mL
1 cup	water	250 mL
2 tsp	cider vinegar	10 mL
2 tbsp	vegetable oil	25 mL
2	eggs	2
2	egg whites	2

1. In a large bowl or plastic bag, combine rice flour, potato starch, tapioca starch, milk powder, sugar, xanthan gum, yeast and salt. Mix well and set aside.

2. In a separate bowl, using a heavy-duty electric mixer with paddle attachment, combine water, vinegar, oil, eggs and egg whites until well blended.

3. With the mixer on lowest speed, slowly add the dry ingredients until combined. With a rubber spatula, scrape the bottom and sides of the bowl. With the mixer on medium speed, beat for 4 minutes.

4. Spoon into prepared pan. Let rise, uncovered, in a warm, draft-free place for 60 to 75 minutes or until the dough has risen to the top of the pan. Meanwhile, preheat oven to 350°F (180°C). Bake for 35 to 45 minutes or until the loaf sounds hollow when tapped on the bottom.

Delicious Desserts

*The perfect ending to any meal! Fresh fruits in season
are the inspiration for several recipes. Choose
the fruit combination to suit your taste.*

～ Traveling with a ～ Gluten Intolerance

- Take extra time to plan any trips, so that they will be more enjoyable and free from stress and worry. When making flight reservations, inform the travel agent of your gluten intolerance. If a meal is to be provided during the flight, advise the agent of your gluten-free dietary needs.

- Pack your own gluten-free bread, cookies or muffins when you travel. Take along your own condiments in your carry-on baggage so they arrive with you. There are lots of ways to do this conveniently. For instance, pack in hard-sided containers that won't be crushed in your luggage or carry-on baggage. Use stackable containers then, when empty, stack them inside each other for compact carrying on the trip home. Your onboard lunch can be packed in a small, collapsible insulated cooler tucked in a corner of your carry-on bag.

- Carry extra baked goods, wrapped in individual servings in airtight containers, in your suitcase.

- Take along fresh fruit and vegetables for snacks during the flight. Include cubes of cheese and gluten-free crackers as the protein and fat take longer to digest and help with hunger during short delays when no other food may be available.

- Before traveling, bake breads or quick breads in two smaller pans $4\frac{1}{2}$-by $2\frac{1}{2}$-inches (250 mL) or $5\frac{3}{4}$-by $3\frac{1}{4}$-inches (500 mL). Bake for 30 to 45 minutes or until done. The smaller-size loaves are more convenient to carry.

- A letter from your doctor explaining your special diet and your need to carry your own food may help avoid problems that stem from carrying food across international borders. Arrive early at the airport and be prepared for a long wait that your special diet may cause.

- Carry a restaurant allergy identification card to present to your server and kitchen staff. You can make your own and laminate it. It is a good idea to make several at the same time as they are easy to lose. When traveling to countries where English is not the first language, have the card translated before you go.

- Hotels may store foods in their freezer for you or you could request a room with a small refrigerator with freezer compartment. Call ahead to make arrangements.

Baked Cheesecake

Decadent, delicious and delightful — need we say more?

TIP
Leave the cheesecake in the oven for 30 minutes after turning the oven off. This helps prevent large cracks.
Be sure to set the timer, as it is easy to forget.

VARIATIONS
Substitute an equal amount of shortbread cookie crumbs from Sue's Shortbread (see recipe, page 164) for the cake crumbs in the base.

∾

Substitute a lower-fat but not whipped or spreadable cream cheese.

∾

Cake crumbs easily if it is slightly frozen.

Preheat oven to 350°F (180°C)
10-inch (25 cm) springform pan, lightly greased

BASE

¼ cup	melted butter	50 mL
¼ cup	packed brown sugar	50 mL
3 cups	White Cake crumbs (see recipe, page 142)	750 mL

CHEESECAKE

2	packages (each 8 oz/250 g) cream cheese, softened	2
1 cup	granulated sugar	250 mL
2 tbsp	cornstarch	25 mL
1 tsp	freshly squeezed lemon juice	5 mL
4	eggs	4
1 cup	milk	250 mL

1. *Base:* In a large bowl, combine butter, brown sugar and cake crumbs. Mix well. Press into prepared pan. Set aside.

2. *Cheesecake:* In a large bowl, using an electric mixer, beat the cream cheese until smooth. Slowly add sugar, cornstarch and lemon juice. Beat until light and fluffy. Add eggs, one at a time, beating well after each. Mix in milk. Pour over the base.

3. Bake in preheated oven for 45 to 55 minutes or until the center is just set. Let cool in oven for 30 minutes with the oven turned off (see Tip, left). Let cool in pan on rack for 30 minutes before refrigerating. Refrigerate until chilled, about 3 hours. Keeps for up to 2 days in the refrigerator.

Double Chocolate Cheesecake with Raspberry Coulis

SERVES 8 TO 10

Chocolate and raspberry are two flavors that go together naturally. Who can resist a sliver of cheesecake served with extra fresh raspberries in season?

TIP

Cheesecake can be frozen for up to 6 weeks. Serve frozen or thaw it in the refrigerator overnight.

Preheat oven to 350°F (180°C)
10-inch (25 cm) springform pan, lightly greased

BASE

2 cups	Fudgy Brownie crumbs (see recipe, page 168)	500 mL

CHEESECAKE

2	packages (each 8 oz/250 g) cream cheese, softened	2
2/3 cup	granulated sugar	150 mL
2 tbsp	sorghum flour	25 mL
3	eggs	3
1 tsp	vanilla extract	5 mL
1 cup	plain yogurt	250 mL
8 oz	semi-sweet chocolate, melted (see Chocolate, page 178)	250 g

RASPBERRY COULIS

1	package (15 oz/425 g) frozen sweetened raspberries, thawed and juice reserved	1

VARIATIONS

Substitute an equal
amount of Chocolate
Fudge Cake (see recipe,
page 140) for the
Fudgy Brownie.

∾

For a less tangy
cheesecake, substitute
whipping cream
for the yogurt.

1. *Base:* Press brownie crumbs onto the bottom of prepared pan. Bake in preheated oven for 10 minutes. Set aside to cool at room temperature.

2. *Cheesecake:* In a large bowl, using an electric mixer, beat the cream cheese until smooth. Slowly add the sugar and sorghum flour. Beat until light and fluffy. Add eggs, one at a time, beating well after each. Add vanilla extract. Fold in yogurt and melted chocolate. Pour over the cooled base.

3. Increase oven temperature to 450°F (230°C). Bake in preheated oven for 10 minutes. Then reduce oven temperature to 250°F (120°C) and continue baking for 35 to 40 minutes or until the center is just set. Let cool in oven for 30 minutes with oven off. Let cool in pan on rack for 30 minutes before refrigerating. Refrigerate until chilled, about 3 hours. Keeps for up to 2 days in the refrigerator.

4. *Raspberry Coulis:* In a food processor or blender, purée thawed raspberries with juice. Press through a fine sieve. Spoon the purée onto individual serving plates. Top with a wedge of cheesecake.

Banana-Pecan Sticky Buns

Thought you'd never be able to enjoy sticky buns again? Well, think again. These are for you.

TIP

We baked this recipe using two types of baking pans. The heavy dark pan baked in the stated time, while the lightweight lighter-colored pan almost burned and the topping hardened on cooling. Adjust baking time according to your baking pan. (See Choosing Your Baking Pans, page 12.)

VARIATION

This recipe can be doubled and baked in two 8-inch (2 L) square baking pans or a single 13-by 9-inch (3 L) baking pan, increasing the baking time by 15 minutes for the large pan.

Preheat oven to 375°F (190°C)
8-inch (2 L) square baking pan, ungreased

²/₃ cup	sorghum flour	150 mL
¹/₂ cup	rice flour	125 mL
¹/₃ cup	potato starch	75 mL
¹/₄ cup	tapioca starch	50 mL
2 tsp	xanthan gum	10 mL
2 tsp	bread machine or instant yeast	10 mL
1¹/₄ tsp	salt	6 mL
1 tsp	ground cinnamon	5 mL
¹/₄ cup	water	50 mL
³/₄ cup	mashed banana	175 mL
¹/₄ cup	liquid honey	50 mL
1 tsp	cider vinegar	5 mL
¹/₄ cup	butter, softened	50 mL
2	eggs	2

PAN GLAZE

¹/₃ cup	melted butter	75 mL
¹/₃ cup	packed brown sugar	75 mL
¹/₃ cup	corn syrup	75 mL
¹/₂ cup	pecan halves	125 mL
¹/₂ cup	raisins	125 mL

BREAD MACHINE METHOD

1. In a large bowl or plastic bag, combine sorghum flour, rice flour, potato starch, tapioca starch, xanthan gum, yeast, salt and cinnamon. Mix well and set aside.

2. Pour water, banana, honey, vinegar, butter and eggs into the bread machine baking pan. Select the Dough Cycle. Allow the liquids to mix until combined.

3. Gradually add the dry ingredients as the bread machine is mixing, scraping with a rubber spatula while adding. Try to incorporate all the dry ingredients within 1 to 2 minutes. Allow the bread machine to complete the cycle.

MIXER METHOD

1. In a large bowl or plastic bag, combine sorghum flour, rice flour, potato starch, tapioca starch, xanthan gum, yeast, salt and cinnamon. Mix well and set aside.

2. In a large bowl, using a heavy-duty mixer with paddle attachment, beat water, banana, honey, vinegar, butter and eggs until well blended.

3. With the mixer on lowest speed, slowly add the dry ingredients until combined. With a rubber spatula, scrape the bottom and sides of the bowl. With the mixer on medium speed, beat for 4 minutes.

FOR BOTH METHODS

4. *Pan Glaze*: In baking pan, combine melted butter, brown sugar and corn syrup. Sprinkle with pecans and raisins. Drop the soft dough by nine heaping spoonfuls on top of the pan glaze. Do not smooth tops. Let rise in a warm, draft-free place for 40 to 50 minutes or until the dough has almost doubled in volume. Bake in preheated oven for 30 to 40 minutes or until sticky buns sound hollow when tapped on the top. Immediately invert pan over a serving platter. Allow to stand for 1 to 2 minutes before removing pan. Serve warm.

Cranberry-Apple Küchen

SERVES 6 TO 8

Best served the day it is made! Start with a buttery-almond crust, then add tangy cranberries and a tart cooking apple.

TIPS

For ease of spreading the dough in the pan, keep dipping the metal spoon in a glass of water.

∾

Use the cranberries directly from the freezer — no need to thaw them.

∾

If almond flour is not readily available, make your own (see Nut Flour, page 180).

Preheat oven to 350°F (180°C)
10-inch (25 cm) springform pan, lightly greased

CRUST

½ cup	sorghum flour	125 mL
¼ cup	cornstarch	50 mL
¼ cup	tapioca starch	50 mL
¼ cup	sweet rice flour	50 mL
¼ cup	almond flour	50 mL
1 tsp	xanthan gum	5 mL
½ tsp	baking soda	2 mL
¼ tsp	salt	1 mL
½ cup	butter, softened	125 mL
½ cup	granulated sugar	125 mL
¼ cup	plain yogurt	50 mL
1	egg yolk	1
½ cup	sliced almonds	125 mL

FILLING

4 cups	sliced apples	1 L
2 cups	cranberries, fresh or frozen	500 mL
¼ cup	granulated sugar	50 mL
2 tbsp	arrowroot starch	25 mL
1 tsp	ground cinnamon	5 mL
¼ cup	sliced almonds	50 mL

GLAZE

⅓ cup	crabapple jelly	75 mL
2 tbsp	water	25 mL

Substitute ½ tsp
(2 mL) of any sweet
spice for the cinnamon.
Try cloves, allspice
or nutmeg.

∽

Choose any fruit
combination you like.
Depending on the fruit,
only 5 cups (1.25 L)
may be needed to
fill the crust.
Try peaches and
blueberries, strawberries
and rhubarb or apples
and raspberries.

∽

Cornstarch can be
substituted for
arrowroot.

1. *Crust:* In a large bowl or plastic bag, combine sorghum flour, cornstarch, tapioca starch, sweet rice flour, almond flour, xanthan gum, baking soda and salt. Mix well and set aside.

2. In a large bowl, using an electric mixer, cream butter and sugar. Beat in yogurt and egg yolk. Stir in dry ingredients. Mix just until blended. Stir in almonds.

3. Using the back of a moistened metal spoon, spread dough evenly on the bottom of and ¾ inches (2 cm) up the side of prepared pan. Let stand for 30 minutes before baking.

4. *Filling:* In a large bowl, toss apples, cranberries, sugar, arrowroot starch and cinnamon. Pour the fruit mixture into the crust, heaping the fruit in the center, leaving the rim of crust exposed. Sprinkle almonds on the rim of the crust.

5. Bake in preheated oven for 60 to 80 minutes or until the crust edge is golden brown and fruit is tender. Let cool in the pan on a rack.

6. *Glaze:* In a small saucepan, bring crabapple jelly and water to a boil, whisking constantly. Reduce heat and boil gently for 4 to 5 minutes or until thickened, whisking occasionally. Brush over fruit. Chill before serving. Keeps for up to 2 days in the refrigerator.

Cherry Clafouti

Friends drop in at dinnertime? Serve this easy-to-prepare custard pudding warm from the oven.

TIP
This is just as delicious served cold the next day.

VARIATION
Omit sugar, if you want to use sweet cherries instead of the sour. If you're using frozen cherries, thaw them first. If using sour cherries from a jar, drain off juices before measuring.

Preheat oven to 400°F (200°C)
8-cup (2 L) oval or square baking dish, lightly greased

3 cups	pitted sour cherries	750 mL
1/4 cup	granulated sugar	50 mL
1/3 cup	rice flour	75 mL
2 tbsp	tapioca starch	25 mL
1/2 tsp	xanthan gum	2 mL
Pinch	salt	Pinch
1 cup	milk	250 mL
1 tbsp	butter	15 mL
2	eggs	2
1/3 cup	granulated sugar	75 mL
1 tsp	vanilla extract	5 mL

1. Combine cherries and 1/4 cup (50 mL) sugar in the bottom of prepared baking dish. Set aside.

2. In a small bowl, combine rice flour, tapioca starch, xanthan gum and salt. Mix well and set aside.

3. In a small saucepan, heat milk and butter over medium heat until tiny bubbles form around the edge. Mix well and set aside.

4. In a large bowl, using an electric mixer, beat eggs and 1/3 cup (75 mL) sugar until light and fluffy. Gradually beat in dry ingredients until smooth. Blend in milk mixture and vanilla extract. Pour over cherries.

5. Bake in preheated oven for 30 to 35 minutes, until puffed and slightly golden. Serve hot.

Creamy Rice Pudding

SERVES 4

As far as we're concerned, this is the ultimate in comfort foods.

TIP

For an extra-creamy pudding, choose short-grain rice.

VARIATIONS

Substitute brown rice for the short-grain white and increase cooking time by 45 minutes. And increase milk to 2½ cups (625 mL).

❧

Substitute cinnamon for nutmeg and dates for raisins.

2 cups	milk	500 mL
⅓ cup	short-grain rice (see Tip, left)	75 mL
3 tbsp	granulated sugar	45 mL
2 tsp	butter	10 mL
Pinch	salt	Pinch
½ tsp	vanilla extract	2 mL
¼ tsp	ground nutmeg	1 mL
⅓ cup	raisins	75 mL

1. In a large saucepan over medium heat, combine milk, rice, sugar, butter and salt. Heat, stirring often, until tiny bubbles form around the edge. Reduce heat to low. Cover and simmer, stirring occasionally, for 1 hour or until rice is tender. Remove from heat. Stir in vanilla, nutmeg and raisins. Serve warm or chilled.

Lemon Sponge Pudding

SERVES 4 TO 6

Whether you remember this as Lemon Cups, Lemon Pudding or Lemon Sponge Pudding, it's still a heavenly light soufflé-like pudding on top with a rich lemony custard sauce beneath.

TIP

It is worth the time to squeeze lemons for freshly squeezed lemon juice. Don't eliminate the zest.

VARIATION

Substitute orange or lime or a combination of both for the lemon.

Preheat oven to 325°F (160°C)
8-cup (2 L) casserole, greased

1 cup	granulated sugar	250 mL
¼ cup	sweet rice flour	50 mL
½ tsp	xanthan gum	2 mL
2 tbsp	vegetable oil	25 mL
Pinch	salt	Pinch
2 tsp	lemon zest	10 mL
⅓ cup	freshly squeezed lemon juice	75 mL
1½ cups	milk	375 mL
3	egg yolks	3
3	egg whites, stiffly beaten	3

1. In a bowl, combine sugar, sweet rice flour, xanthan gum, oil, salt, lemon zest and juice. Set aside.

2. In a small saucepan, heat milk over medium heat until tiny bubbles form around the edge. Set aside.

3. In a separate large bowl, using an electric mixer, beat egg yolks until light and fluffy. Blend in milk and lemon mixture. Fold in beaten egg whites. Pour into prepared casserole.

4. Place casserole in a larger pan. Pour boiling water into the larger pan to reach half way up the sides of the casserole. Bake in preheated oven for 40 minutes or until the top is set and cake is slightly golden. Serve warm or chilled.

Harvest Caramel

Pumpkin, maple syrup and spices add a delicious twist to a classic dessert.

TIP

Using a pastry brush dipped in water, occasionally brush down any sugar crystals that appear on the side of the pan while heating the sugar.

VARIATION

Use cooked, puréed winter squash for the pumpkin.

Preheat oven to 350°F (180°C)
Seven individual heatproof ramekins or custard cups

CARAMEL

1 cup	granulated sugar	250 mL
1/4 cup	water	50 mL
1/8 tsp	freshly squeezed lemon juice	0.5 mL

CUSTARD

8	egg yolks	8
1/2 cup	pure maple syrup	125 mL
1 1/2 cups	pumpkin purée (not pie filling)	375 mL
1/2 tsp	ground cinnamon	2 mL
1/2 tsp	ground ginger	2 mL
Pinch	ground allspice	Pinch
Pinch	ground nutmeg	Pinch
2 cups	half-and-half (10%) cream	500 mL

1. *Caramel:* In a heavy saucepan over low heat, dissolve sugar in water. Add lemon juice. Without stirring, cook over medium heat until mixture begins to boil. Continue to cook until mixture turns a deep caramel brown. Remove from heat immediately, as mixture continues to cook. Pour into cups.

2. *Custard:* In a large bowl, using an electric mixer, beat egg yolks with maple syrup. Add pumpkin and spices and mix until blended.

3. Heat cream over medium heat until tiny bubbles form around the edge. Stirring constantly, gradually add cream to the pumpkin mixture. Divide evenly among custard cups.

4. Place custard cups in a larger pan. Pour boiling water into the larger pan to reach half way up the sides of the custard cups. Bake in preheated oven for 30 minutes or until knife blade inserted near the center comes out clean. Remove cups from hot water. Let stand for 30 minutes. Refrigerate until serving for up to one week. If desired, turn custards out onto individual serving plates.

Gingerbread

SERVES 9

A tangy lemon sauce is what turns this traditional gingerbread into something special. In fact, to make sure you don't run out, we suggest that you double the Lotsa Lemon Sauce (see recipe, page 130).

TIP

The batter thickens during the standing time before baking. Allowing the batter to stand results in a more tender cake.

VARIATIONS

Substitute potato starch for the tapioca.

Add ½ cup (125 mL) sunflower seeds to the batter.

Preheat oven to 350°F (180°C)
8-inch (2 L) square baking pan, lightly greased

1 cup	boiling water	250 mL
½ cup	shortening	125 mL
¾ cup	whole bean flour	175 mL
¾ cup	sorghum flour	175 mL
¼ cup	tapioca starch	50 mL
1 tsp	xanthan gum	5 mL
½ tsp	GF baking powder	2 mL
¼ tsp	baking soda	1 mL
¼ tsp	salt	1 mL
1½ tsp	ground ginger	7 mL
¾ tsp	ground cinnamon	4 mL
2	eggs	2
⅔ cup	fancy molasses	150 mL
⅔ cup	granulated sugar	150 mL
	Lotsa Lemon Sauce	

1. In a small bowl, pour boiling water over shortening. Set aside to melt and cool slightly.

2. In a large bowl, sift together whole bean flour, sorghum flour, tapioca starch, xanthan gum, baking powder, baking soda, salt, ginger and cinnamon. Resift and set aside.

3. In a separate bowl, using an electric mixer, beat eggs, molasses and sugar. Add shortening mixture and beat until smooth. Stir in dry ingredients. Mix just until blended. Pour into prepared pan. Let stand for 30 minutes before baking.

4. Bake in preheated oven for 45 to 55 minutes or until a cake tester inserted in the center comes out clean. Let cool in the pan on a rack for 10 minutes. Remove from the pan and serve warm with Lotsa Lemon Sauce.

Summertime Trifle

SERVES 4 TO 6

6-cup (1.5 L) clear glass bowl or individual serving dishes

> *Trifle is a traditional English dessert that looks spectacular layered in a large glass bowl. It is a lifesaver when you have to feed a crowd, and everyone loves it. Our version features citrus to contrast with sweet, colorful fruit and the velvet creaminess of custard.*

3 tbsp	cornstarch	45 mL
1/3 cup	granulated sugar	75 mL
2 cups	milk	500 mL
3	egg yolks	3
1/2 tsp	almond extract	2 mL
1/4	White Cake, cut into 3/4-inch (2 cm) cubes, (see recipe, page 142)	1/4
2 to 3 tbsp	orange-flavored liqueur	25 to 45 mL
3 cups	fresh fruit (see Variations, left)	750 mL
1/4 cup	toasted sliced almonds (see Nuts, page 180)	50 mL

TIPS

If custard boils after the eggs are added, it curdles. Watch carefully!

∽

Custard can be covered with waxed paper or plastic wrap placed directly on the surface and refrigerated for up to 1 day.

VARIATIONS

Choose pears and cranberries; blackberries, raspberries or a mixture of berries; or stewed rhubarb and strawberries. Garnish with whipped cream, if desired.

∽

We found that an angel food cake didn't absorb enough liqueur when it replaced the white cake.

MICROWAVE METHOD

1. In a large bowl, combine cornstarch and sugar. Add milk. Microwave on High for 5 to 6 minutes or until steaming, stirring every 2 minutes. Whisk about one-third of hot milk mixture into egg yolks. Gradually whisk yolk into remaining milk mixture and microwave on High for 1 to 2 minutes or until bubbly around the edge. Do not let boil. Stir in almond extract. Set aside to cool.

STOVE-TOP METHOD

1. In a saucepan, combine cornstarch and sugar. Add milk. Heat over medium for 5 to 6 minutes or until steaming, stirring constantly. Whisk about one-third of hot milk mixture into egg yolks. Gradually whisk yolk mixture into remaining milk mixture and return to heat for 3 to 5 minutes or until thick. Do not let boil. Stir in almond extract. Set aside to cool.

FOR BOTH METHODS

2. In a large serving bowl, line the bottom and sides with cake cubes. Sprinkle with liqueur. Spread half of custard over the cake. Spread with fruit and top with remaining custard. Chill for at least 1 hour or up to 8 hours. Garnish with toasted almond slices.

Three-Fruit Cobbler

SERVES 6 TO 8

This cobbler is a variation of the famous Nova Scotia dessert, blueberry grunt, but without the blueberries. It brings together our favorite summertime fruits — peaches, plums and pears.

TIPS

See tips for Biscuits and Cobblers, page 62.

◆

We suggest a deep casserole dish so the cobbler doesn't boil over onto your clean oven.

◆

No need to peel the tender fruit — the skins soften as the cobbler bakes.

◆

For best results, fruit should be perfectly ripe. If necessary, ripen fruit in a paper bag on the counter until fragrant and it yields to gentle pressure.

Preheat oven to 400°F (200°C)
Deep 8-cup (2 L) casserole dish

COBBLER BISCUIT

1 cup	soy flour	250 mL
2/3 cup	brown rice flour	150 mL
1/4 cup	tapioca starch	50 mL
1/4 cup	granulated sugar	50 mL
1 tsp	xanthan gum	5 mL
1 1/2 tsp	GF baking powder	7 mL
1/2 tsp	baking soda	2 mL
1/4 tsp	salt	1 mL
1/3 cup	cold butter, cut into 1-inch (2.5 cm) cubes	75 mL
2/3 cup	buttermilk	150 mL

BASE

1/3 cup	granulated sugar	75 mL
1 tbsp	cornstarch	15 mL
2 cups	coarsely chopped peaches or nectarines, about 3 medium	500 mL
2 cups	coarsely chopped pears, about 3 medium	500 mL
2 cups	coarsely chopped plums, about 4 large	500 mL
1 tbsp	freshly squeezed lemon juice	15 mL

1. *Cobbler Biscuit:* In a large bowl, sift together soy flour, brown rice flour, tapioca starch, sugar, xanthan gum, baking powder, baking soda and salt. Using a pastry blender or two knives, cut in butter until mixture resembles small peas. Add buttermilk all at once, stirring with a fork to make a sticky dough. Let stand for 30 minutes.

Use apples, raspberries and pears (or any other combination of seasonal fruit) to make up to 6 cups (1.5 L) in total.

2. *Base:* In casserole dish, mix together sugar and cornstarch. Gently stir in peaches, pears, plums and lemon juice. Place in preheated oven for 15 minutes or until hot and bubbly.

3. Drop biscuit topping, by heaping tablespoonfuls (15 mL), onto hot bubbly fruit mixture. Bake in preheated oven for 20 to 25 minutes or until top is golden. Serve immediately.

Rhubarb Crisp

SERVES 4 TO 6

Looking for a delicious way to celebrate the first fruit of the season? Here it is.

TIPS

Purchase either gluten-free rice flakes or rolled rice cereal.

For a crisper topping, cover with foil for the first half of the baking time.

VARIATIONS

Substitute thawed, frozen rhubarb for the fresh.

Replace half the rhubarb with the same quantity of sliced, fresh strawberries. Reduce corn syrup to ⅓ cup (75 mL).

Preheat oven to 375°F (190°C)
8-cup (2 L) casserole, lightly greased

TOPPING

½ cup	packed brown sugar	125 mL
½ cup	sorghum flour	125 mL
½ cup	GF rice cereal (see Tips, left)	125 mL
2 tsp	orange zest	10 mL
½ tsp	ground ginger	2 mL
⅓ cup	cold butter, cut into 1-inch (2.5 cm) cubes	75 mL
½ cup	chopped walnuts	125 mL

BASE

½ cup	corn syrup, warmed	125 mL
3 tbsp	cornstarch	45 mL
5 to 6 cups	chopped fresh rhubarb	1.25 to 1.5 L

1. *Topping:* In a bowl, combine brown sugar, sorghum flour, rice cereal, orange zest and ginger. With a pastry blender or two knives, cut in butter until crumbly. Add walnuts. Set aside.

2. *Base:* In prepared casserole, mix corn syrup and cornstarch to form a paste. Add rhubarb and stir until coated. Sprinkle crumb topping over the rhubarb. Do not pack.

3. Bake crisp in preheated oven for 50 minutes or until the rhubarb is tender. Serve warm.

Banana Seed Bread (pages 81 and 97)

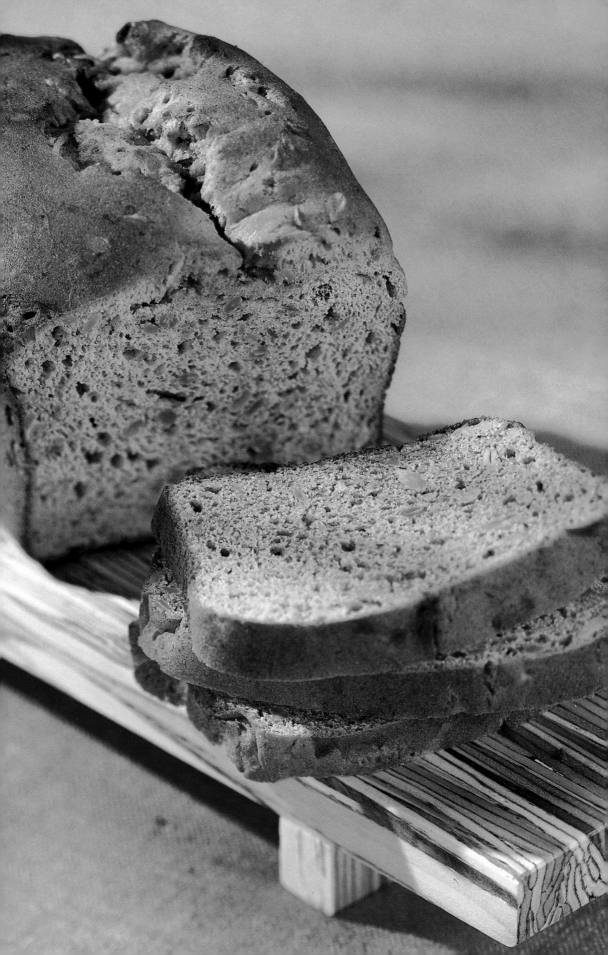

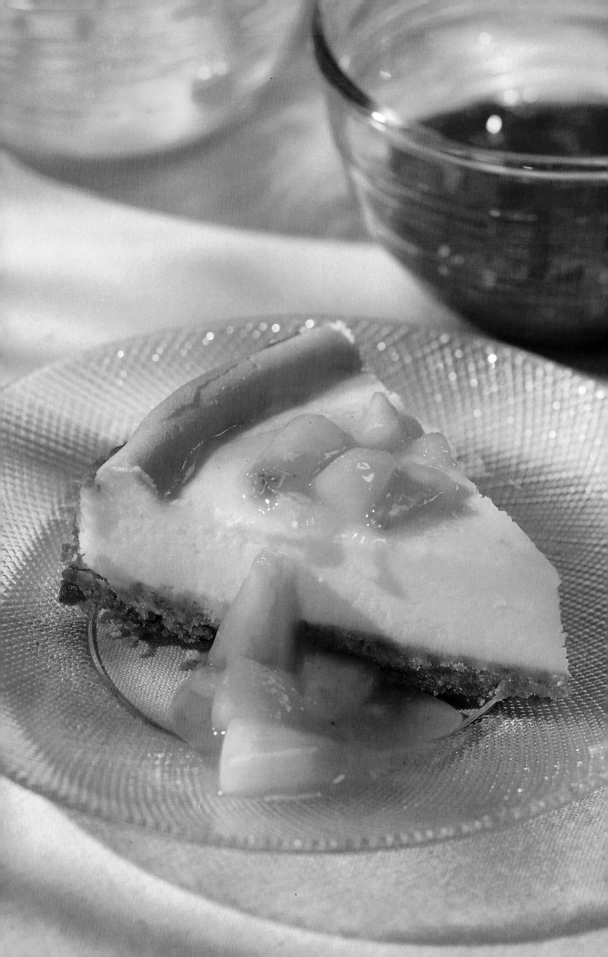

Fresh Peach Dessert Sauce

MAKES 4 CUPS (1 L)

An abundance of peaches in the supermarket inspired this fresh no-cook sauce. Serve over cheesecake or white cake.

VARIATION
Add 1 cup (250 mL) blueberries or coarsely diced plums for a mixed fresh fruit sauce.

4	peaches, peeled and chopped (see Blanch, page 178)	4
¼ cup	granulated sugar	50 mL
½ tsp	freshly squeezed lemon juice	2 mL
2 tbsp	water	25 mL

1. In a bowl, combine peaches, sugar, lemon juice and water. Stir gently to mix. Refrigerate for at least 1 hour.

Raspberry Dessert Sauce

MAKES 2½ CUPS (625 ML)

Mixing fresh and frozen berries gives this sauce a distinct fresh berry flavor. Serve over chocolate or angel food cakes.

TIP
If only unsweetened raspberries are available, add 2 to 3 tbsp (25 to 45 mL) granulated sugar.

2 tbsp	cornstarch	25 mL
1	package (15 oz/425 g) frozen sweetened raspberries, thawed, drained and syrup reserved	1
1 cup	fresh raspberries	250 mL

1. In a large bowl, combine cornstarch and ¾ cup (175 mL) reserved raspberry syrup. Microwave on High, stirring once, for 4 minutes or until thick and shiny or in a saucepan over medium heat on top of the stove, stirring frequently.
2. Gently fold in thawed and fresh raspberries. Refrigerate for 1 hour before serving.

Baked Cheesecake (page 113) with Fresh Peach Dessert Sauce and Raspberry Dessert Sauce (page 129)

Blueberry Dessert Sauce

MAKES 2 CUPS (500 ML)

Enjoy this versatile sauce served over cheesecake, angel food cake or pancakes.

TIP
This sauce is great either warm or cold. Small amounts can be frozen to quickly thaw when guests arrive.

2 tbsp	cornstarch	25 mL
1/3 cup	granulated sugar	75 mL
3 cups	frozen blueberries, thawed and drained, juice reserved	750 mL
2 tbsp	freshly squeezed lemon juice	25 mL

1. In a saucepan combine cornstarch and sugar. Slowly add 1/3 cup (75 mL) reserved blueberry juice and lemon juice, stirring constantly. Add blueberries. Cook and stir over medium heat until mixture boils and becomes thick and shiny. Cool, stirring occasionally. Sauce keeps for up to 2 weeks in the refrigerator.

Lotsa Lemon Sauce

MAKES 1½ CUPS (375 ML)

Not too tangy, not too sweet, just perfect! Any excuse is a good excuse to make this recipe frequently.

TIP
Try this lemon sauce drizzled over Gingered Pumpkin Snacking Cake (see recipe, page 150) and Gingerbread (see recipe, page 124).

1/2 cup	granulated sugar	125 mL
3 tbsp	cornstarch	45 mL
1 1/3 cups	water	325 mL
2 tsp	lemon zest	10 mL
1/3 cup	freshly squeezed lemon juice	75 mL
3 tbsp	butter	45 mL

MICROWAVE METHOD

1. In a bowl, mix together sugar and cornstarch. Add water, lemon zest, lemon juice and butter. Microwave on High, stirring once or twice, for 3 to 5 minutes or until it boils and thickens.

STOVE-TOP METHOD

1. In a saucepan, combine sugar and cornstarch. Add water, lemon zest, lemon juice and butter. Heat over medium for 5 to 8 minutes or until it boils and thickens, stirring constantly. Set aside to cool.

Pies and Cakes

There's no need to wait for a birthday or anniversary to serve a special cake or pie. Enjoy a slice with a cup of tea or coffee or, better yet, a cold glass of milk.

～ Pastry Making Tips ～

- We provide directions for both the food processor and the traditional methods of making pastry. The food processor method is easier to mix without over-handling. Process the ingredients, by pulsing, until the dough begins to stick together. With your fingertips, gather the dough into a light ball and gently press together.

- In the traditional method, when using a pastry blender or two knives to cut in the shortening or butter, cut only until the pieces are the size of small peas. This results in a tender, flaky pastry. If too finely cut in or mashed, the pastry tends to be tough and heavy.

- Form enough dough to make one shell into a round, flattened disk. This shape is easier to roll out into the circle for a pie plate.

- Refrigerate the dough, tightly wrapped, for at least 1 hour before rolling out. It can be left in the refrigerator up to 3 days or in the freezer for 3 months.

- Roll out the dough between two sheets of waxed paper — it is easier to handle. Or, generously flour a wooden board and rolling pin with sweet rice flour. Re-flour the board and rolling pin occasionally to prevent sticking.

- Roll out the dough using light, long strokes from the center to the edges. Roll out to each side, then back to the center. Repeat until the dough is 1-inch (2.5 cm) larger than the pie plate. It should be about $1/4$ inch (0.5 cm) thick.

- Ease the pastry into the pie plate. Do not worry if it breaks where it touches the rim of the plate. Just patch the shell with pastry scraps.

Peachy Plum Hazelnut Galette

SERVES 8 TO 12

Simpler than pie but with all the same homemade goodness, this galette makes excellent use of an abundance of summer fruits.

TIPS

If hazelnut flour is not readily available in your area, make your own from hazelnuts (see Nut Flour, page 180).

❧

The jelly spreads more evenly when microwaved on High for 20 seconds.

VARIATION

Prepare the pastry with almond flour and sprinkle the prepared galette with sliced almonds. Almonds toast as the galette bakes.

Preheat oven to 425°F (220°C)
Large baking sheet, generously dusted with sweet rice flour

1	Hazelnut Pastry (see recipe, page 134)	1
3 cups	peeled, sliced peaches, about 5 medium	750 mL
2 cups	sliced red or purple plums, about 4 large	500 mL
¼ cup	hazelnut flour (see Tips, left)	50 mL
¼ cup	granulated sugar	50 mL
2 tbsp	cornstarch	25 mL
1 tbsp	butter	15 mL
⅓ cup	chopped hazelnuts	75 mL
1 tbsp	granulated sugar	15 mL
2 tbsp	grape or red currant jelly (see Tips, left)	25 mL

1. Place the chilled Hazelnut Pastry disk in the center of prepared pan. Cover with waxed paper and roll out to a 12-inch (30 cm) circle.

2. In a large bowl, lightly toss together peaches, plums, hazelnut flour, ¼ cup (50 mL) sugar and cornstarch. Set aside.

3. Carefully remove the waxed paper. Place the fruit mixture on pastry to within 2 inches (5 cm) of the edge. Dot with butter and sprinkle with hazelnuts. Carefully fold the pastry up over the filling to form a ragged edge, leaving fruit exposed in the center. Sprinkle pastry with 1 tbsp (15 mL) sugar.

4. Bake in preheated oven for 15 minutes. Reduce heat to 375°F (190°C) and bake for 25 to 30 minutes longer or until fruit is tender and pastry is lightly browned. Brush with jelly.

Hazelnut Pastry

**MAKES 1
SINGLE-CRUST
9-INCH (23 CM) PIE**

*Quick and easy,
shortbread tender and
simple to serve — no
need to wait for the
holidays or special
occasions to enjoy the
hazelnut flavor. We use
Hazelnut Pastry for
fruit, pumpkin and
cream pies.*

TIPS

This recipe can be
doubled or tripled
but leave salt at
¼ tsp (1 mL).

∽

For a pre-baked pie
shell, prick bottom
and sides of shell with
a fork before baking.

∽

Work quickly to keep
the pastry cold and to
prevent the butter
from softening.

∽

If hazelnut flour is
not readily available,
make your own (see
Nut Flour, page 180).

3 tbsp	ice water	45 mL
1 tsp	cider vinegar	5 mL
1	egg yolk	1
½ cup	sorghum flour	125 mL
¼ cup	cornstarch	50 mL
¼ cup	tapioca starch	50 mL
¼ cup	sweet rice flour	50 mL
¼ cup	hazelnut flour (see Tips, left)	50 mL
1 tsp	xanthan gum	5 mL
¼ tsp	salt	1 mL
½ cup	cold butter, cut into 1-inch (2.5 cm) cubes	125 mL

FOOD PROCESSOR METHOD

1. In a small bowl, combine ice water, vinegar and egg yolk. Set aside.

2. In a food processor fitted with a metal blade, pulse sorghum flour, cornstarch, tapioca starch, sweet rice flour, hazelnut flour, xanthan gum and salt until mixed.

3. Add butter. Pulse until mixture resembles small peas, about 5 to 10 seconds. With machine running, add egg yolk mixture in a slow steady stream. Process until dough just holds together. Do not let it form a ball.

TRADITIONAL METHOD

1. In a small bowl, combine ice water, vinegar and egg yolk. Set aside.

2. In a large bowl, sift sorghum flour, cornstarch, tapioca starch, sweet rice flour, hazelnut flour, xanthan gum and salt. Resift.

3. Using a pastry blender or two knives, cut in butter until mixture resembles small peas. Stirring with a fork, sprinkle egg yolk mixture, a little at a time, over the flour-butter mixture to make soft dough.

VARIATION

Substitute pecan flour or almond flour for hazelnut flour.

FOR BOTH METHODS

4. Gently gather dough into a ball and place on plastic wrap and flatten into a disk. Wrap well. Refrigerate for at least 1 hour.

5. Place the pastry disk between two sheets of waxed paper. Gently, with quick, light strokes of the rolling pin, roll out the pastry dough into a circle 1 inch (2.5 cm) larger than the diameter of the pie plate. Carefully remove the top sheet of waxed paper. Invert the pastry over the pie plate, easing it in. Carefully remove the remaining sheet of waxed paper.

6. Trim excess pastry to edge of pie plate and patch any cracks with trimmings. Press edge with a fork. For a more attractive finish, using a sharp knife, trim the edge evenly, leaving a 1-inch (2.5 cm) overhang. Tuck pastry under to form a raised double rim. Flute or crimp the edges.

7. *To bake unfilled pastry shell:* To prevent pastry from shrinking or puffing up, prick bottom and sides with a fork. Bake at 425°F (220°C) for 18 to 20 minutes or until golden. Let cool completely before filling.

8. *To bake filled pastry shell:* Do not prick. Spoon the filling into unbaked pastry shell and bake according to individual recipe directions.

Pie Pastry

Easy as pie — truer words were never spoken and making pie becomes easier each time you do it. We'd like to say that this is truly a no-fail pastry.

TIP

Recipe can be doubled or tripled but leave salt at 1/2 tsp (2 mL).

VARIATION

This can be made into tart shells to fill with custard and fresh fruit.

1/3 cup	ice water	75 mL
2 tsp	cider vinegar	10 mL
2	egg yolks	2
1 cup	rice flour	250 mL
1 cup	cornstarch	250 mL
1/2 cup	tapioca starch	125 mL
2 tsp	xanthan gum	10 mL
1/4 tsp	salt	1 mL
1 cup	shortening, softened	250 mL

FOOD PROCESSOR METHOD

1. In a small bowl, combine ice water, vinegar and egg yolks. Set aside.
2. In a food processor fitted with a metal blade, pulse rice flour, cornstarch, tapioca starch, xanthan gum and salt until mixed.
3. Add shortening and pulse until mixture resembles small peas, about 5 to 10 seconds. With machine running, add egg yolk mixture in a slow steady stream. Process until dough just holds together. Do not let it form a ball.

TRADITIONAL METHOD

1. In a small bowl, combine ice water, vinegar and egg yolks. Set aside.
2. In a large bowl, sift rice flour, cornstarch, tapioca starch, xanthan gum and salt. Resift.
3. Using a pastry blender or two knives, cut in shortening until mixture resembles small peas. Stirring with a fork, sprinkle egg yolk mixture, a little at a time, over the flour-shortening mixture to make soft dough.

FOR BOTH METHODS

4. Divide dough in half. Gently gather dough into a ball and place each half on plastic wrap and flatten into a disk and wrap well. Refrigerate for at least 1 hour. Let cold pastry stand for 10 minutes at room temperature before rolling out.

5. Place the pastry disk between two sheets of waxed paper. Gently, with quick, light strokes of the rolling pin, roll out the pastry dough into a circle 1 inch (2.5 cm) larger than the diameter of the pie plate. Carefully remove the top sheet of waxed paper. Invert the pastry over the pie plate, easing it in. Carefully remove the remaining sheet of waxed paper.

6. Trim excess pastry to edge of pie plate and patch any cracks with trimmings. Press edge with a fork. For a more attractive finish, using a sharp knife, trim the edge evenly, leaving a 1-inch (2.5 cm) overhang. Tuck pastry under to form a raised double rim. Flute or crimp the edges.

7. *To bake unfilled pastry shell*: To prevent pastry from shrinking or puffing up, prick bottom and sides with a fork. Bake at 425°F (220°C) for 18 to 20 minutes or until golden. Let cool completely before filling.

8. *To bake filled pastry shell*: Do not prick. Spoon the filling into unbaked pastry shell and bake according to individual recipe directions.

Strawberry Mousse Pie

Strawberries, a crowd pleaser, give this a refreshing light taste on a hot summer day.

TIPS

If the filling appears to be too thin, before folding into the beaten evaporated milk, chill in the refrigerator until it molds when dropped from a spoon. This may take up to 30 minutes.

∽

To get maximum volume from the evaporated milk, chill milk, bowl and beaters for at least 30 minutes.

VARIATIONS

Substitute raspberries for the strawberries.

∽

If substituting unsweetened strawberries for the sweetened, increase granulated sugar to ¼ cup (50 mL).

∽

In a hurry? Spoon the strawberry mousse into parfait glasses or a large glass serving bowl.

1	package (¼ oz/7 g) unflavored gelatin	1
¾ cup	orange juice	175 mL
1	package (14 oz/425 g) frozen sweetened strawberries, partially thawed	1
½ cup	chilled evaporated milk	125 mL
2 tbsp	granulated sugar	25 mL
1	baked 9-inch (23 cm) single-crust pie shell (see recipes, pages 134 or 136)	1

1. In a small saucepan, sprinkle gelatin over orange juice. Let stand for 1 minute to soften. Warm over medium heat, whisking constantly, for about 2 minutes or until dissolved.

2. Add partially frozen strawberries and stir until berries are thawed and mixture is consistency of egg whites. Chill if necessary (see Tips, left).

3. In a large bowl, using an electric mixer, beat evaporated milk until soft peaks form. Gradually add sugar, beating until stiff. Slowly add one-quarter of thickened strawberry mixture to beaten evaporated milk, beating constantly. Fold in remaining strawberry mixture. Spoon into baked pastry shell. Refrigerate for at least 3 hours or until set. Garnish with fresh strawberries.

～ Cake Baking Tips ～

- We recommend sifting then resifting the dry ingredients because the batter is mixed very little. If the gluten-free flours and starches lump or are not mixed well, the cake may bake with pockets of these dry ingredients.

- Cake recipes often require creaming the shortening or butter and sugar before adding the eggs. Creaming the butter first, then slowly beating in the sugar improves the texture. Adding the eggs, one at a time, beating after each, results in an even lighter cake.

- Adding the dry and liquid ingredients alternately, mixing just until blended after each, results in a more even-textured cake. This mixing may be done using low speed of the electric mixer or a rubber spatula.

- To lighten baked foods containing eggs, separate the eggs and beat the whites until stiff but not dry and fold them into the batter as the last step before putting the batter into the baking pan.

- Letting the batter stand for 30 minutes at room temperature before baking results in a lighter-textured, more-tender cake. However, if you are short of time, bake the cake immediately.

- There are three ways to tell whether a cake is done: if the top, when pressed lightly, springs back; when a wooden skewer inserted in the center comes out clean; and when the cake just begins to pull away from the pan.

- Unless the recipe recommends differently, let the cake cool for 10 minutes in the pan. Then, using a metal spatula or knife, trace around the edge between the pan and cake and turn it out onto a cooling rack to cool completely before frosting.

- To remove the cake from a springform pan, be sure to loosen the cake from edge of pan before removing the side by opening the clip on the side.

Chocolate Fudge Cake

SERVES 8 TO 10

Susan, a celiac in our neighborhood, cuts our fudge cake into cubes and freezes them. Then when she has a chocolate attack, she can take a piece for a quick treat. The cake tastes just as delicious as it looks on the cover.

TIPS

Sifting the dry ingredients twice helps distribute the cocoa evenly.

∿

It is easier to spread the thick batter to the edges of the pan with a moist rubber spatula.

∿

Refrigerate frosted cake for up to 3 days. Freeze individual layers, wrapped airtight, for up to 1 month.

VARIATION

For a milk chocolate-flavored cake, decrease the unsweetened cocoa powder by 1/4 cup (50 mL) and substitute granulated sugar for the packed brown sugar.

Preheat oven to 350°F (180°C)
Two 8-inch (20 cm) round pans, lightly greased

3/4 cup	whole bean flour	175 mL
3/4 cup	sorghum flour	175 mL
1/2 cup	potato starch	125 mL
1/4 cup	tapioca starch	50 mL
1 tsp	xanthan gum	5 mL
1/2 tsp	GF baking powder	2 mL
1 1/2 tsp	baking soda	7 mL
1/2 tsp	salt	2 mL
3/4 cup	unsweetened cocoa powder	175 mL
3/4 cup	shortening or butter, softened	175 mL
1 1/2 cups	packed brown sugar	375 mL
3	eggs	3
2 tsp	vanilla extract	10 mL
2 cups	GF sour cream	500 mL

1. In a large bowl, sift together whole bean flour, sorghum flour, potato starch, tapioca starch, xanthan gum, baking powder, baking soda, salt and cocoa. Resift and set aside.

2. In a separate bowl, using an electric mixer, cream shortening and brown sugar until light and fluffy. Add eggs, one at a time, beating well after each addition. Stir in vanilla extract. Stir in dry ingredients alternately with sour cream to shortening-sugar mixture, making three additions of dry ingredients and two of sour cream. Stir just until combined after each addition. Spoon into prepared pans. Spread to edges and smooth tops with a moist rubber spatula. Let stand for 30 minutes.

3. Bake in preheated oven for 35 to 45 minutes or until a cake tester inserted in the center comes out clean. Let cakes cool in pans on racks for 10 minutes. Remove from pans and let cool completely on racks. Frost with Orange Frosting (see recipe page 156).

Angel Food Cake

TIPS

This is an ideal time to use liquid egg whites available in cartons. Store the cake at room temperature for up to 3 days or freeze, wrapped airtight, for up to 1 month.

❧

Make sure the mixer bowl, beaters and the tube pan are completely free of grease.

❧

It is easier to separate an egg when it is cold, right from the refrigerator, because the yolk is less apt to break.

VARIATION

Add ¼ cup (50 mL) unsweetened cocoa powder to the dry ingredients to make a Chocolate Angel Food Cake. For a Mocha Angel Food Cake, add 1 tsp (5 mL) of instant coffee granules with the cocoa.

Preheat oven to 350°F (180°C)
10-inch (4 L) tube pan, completely free of grease

½ cup	white rice flour	125 mL
⅓ cup	cornstarch	75 mL
⅓ cup	GF confectioner's (icing) sugar	75 mL
1 tsp	xanthan gum	5 mL
12	eggs whites, warmed to room temperature (see Techniques Glossary, page 178)	12
1 tbsp	freshly squeezed lemon juice	15 mL
1½ tsp	cream of tartar	7 mL
¼ tsp	salt	1 mL
¾ cup	granulated sugar	175 mL
1 tsp	almond extract	5 mL

1. In a small bowl, sift together rice flour, cornstarch, confectioner's sugar and xanthan gum. Resift and set aside.

2. In a separate large bowl, using an electric mixer, beat egg whites until foamy. While beating, add lemon juice, cream of tartar and salt. Continue to beat until egg whites are stiff. Gradually add sugar. Continue to beat until mixture is very stiff and glossy but not dry.

3. Sift dry ingredients, one-quarter at a time, over beaten egg whites. Gently fold in each addition until well blended. Fold in almond extract. Spoon into prepared pan. Run a knife through the batter to remove large air bubbles. Smooth top with a moist rubber spatula.

4. Bake immediately in preheated oven for 30 to 40 minutes or until the cake springs back when lightly touched. Invert pan over a funnel or bottle until completely cooled. Using a spatula, loosen the outside and inside edges of the pan. Remove from pan.

White Cake

Begin with this light, versatile cake to make desserts that are sure to please. We like to use it to make trifle, cupcakes or to top it with fresh fruit.

TIP
Freeze cakes with no icing to use as a crumb base for cheesecakes or to cut into cubes for a trifle. Freeze individual layers, wrapped airtight, for up to 1 month.

VARIATIONS
Double the recipe, except for the salt and baking powder. Bake in a 10-inch (25 cm) springform pan for 75 minutes to make a larger cake for special occasions.

∾

For a quick, easy dessert, smother this cake with warm Chocolate Glaze, (see recipe, page 155).

Preheat oven to 350°F (180°C)
8-inch (2 L) square pan, lightly greased

²⁄₃ cup	white rice flour	150 mL
½ cup	tapioca starch	125 mL
⅓ cup	cornstarch	75 mL
¾ tsp	xanthan gum	4 mL
1½ tsp	GF baking powder	7 mL
½ tsp	salt	2 mL
½ cup	shortening or butter, softened	125 mL
¾ cup	granulated sugar	175 mL
3	eggs	3
¾ tsp	vanilla extract	4 mL
1 tsp	cider vinegar	5 mL
½ cup	milk	125 mL

1. In a large bowl, sift rice flour, tapioca starch, cornstarch, xanthan gum, baking powder and salt. Resift and set aside.

2. In a separate bowl, using an electric mixer, cream shortening and sugar until light and fluffy. Add eggs, one at a time, beating well after each addition. Stir in vanilla extract and vinegar. Stir in dry ingredients alternately with milk, making three additions of dry ingredients and two of milk. Stir just until combined after each addition. Spoon into prepared pan. Spread to edges and smooth top with a moist rubber spatula. Let stand for 30 minutes.

3. Bake in preheated oven for 35 to 40 minutes or until a cake tester inserted in the center comes out clean. Let cool in the pan on a rack for 10 minutes. Remove from the pan and let cool completely on rack.

Peach Upside-Down Cake

TIPS

Purchase sliced peaches packed in juice, not syrup.

∽

The addition of dry ingredients and juice may be done either with the mixer on the lowest speed or with a rubber spatula or wooden spoon.

VARIATIONS

Substitute 4 or 5 medium, fresh peeled peaches for the canned peaches and milk for the juice.

∽

Sprinkle 1/3 to 1/2 cup (75 to 125 mL) fresh blueberries over the peaches before the batter is spooned on.

Preheat oven to 350°F (180°C)
9-inch (2.5 L) square pan, lightly greased

BASE

1/2 cup	apricot jam	125 mL
1	can (28 oz/796 mL) sliced peaches in pear juice, drained (see Tips, left)	1

CAKE

2/3 cup	white rice flour	150 mL
1/2 cup	tapioca starch	125 mL
1/3 cup	cornstarch	75 mL
3/4 tsp	xanthan gum	4 mL
1 1/2 tsp	GF baking powder	7 mL
1/2 tsp	salt	2 mL
1/2 cup	shortening or butter, softened	125 mL
2/3 cup	granulated sugar	150 mL
3	eggs	3
1/4 tsp	almond extract	1 mL

1. *Base:* Drain peaches, reserving 1/2 cup (125 mL) of the juice. Set aside. Spread jam evenly in prepared pan. Arrange peach slices over top.

2. *Cake:* In a large bowl or plastic bag, combine rice flour, tapioca starch, cornstarch, xanthan gum, baking powder and salt. Mix well and set aside.

3. In a separate bowl, using an electric mixer, cream shortening and sugar until light and fluffy. Add eggs, one at a time, beating well after each addition. Stir in almond extract. Stir in dry ingredients alternately with reserved juice, making three additions of dry ingredients and two of juice. Stir just until combined after each addition. Spoon over peaches in prepared pan. Smooth top with a moist rubber spatula. Let stand for 30 minutes.

4. Bake in preheated oven for 45 to 50 minutes or until a cake tester inserted in the center comes out clean. Let cool in the pan on a rack for 5 minutes. Invert the pan over a serving plate. Remove pan and serve warm.

Pineapple-Carrot Cake

SERVES 12 TO 16

This cake is so well loved by everyone that many brides choose it for their wedding cake. The pineapple adds a moist sweetness. Perfect topped with Cream Cheese Frosting (see recipe, page 156).

TIP

Watch for the deep, rich golden color of the soy flour; you may want to tent this cake with foil partway through the baking to slow down the browning. Line the bottom of baking pan with waxed paper to prevent sticking.

VARIATIONS

Substitute desiccated coconut for the walnuts.

∽

If you prefer, bake in a 13-by-9-inch (3 L) baking pan and reduce baking time by approximately 10 to 15 minutes.

Preheat oven to 350°F (180°C)
10-inch (3 L) Bundt pan, lightly greased

1¼ cups	brown rice flour	300 mL
1 cup	soy flour	250 mL
¼ cup	potato starch	50 mL
¼ cup	tapioca starch	50 mL
1 tsp	xanthan gum	5 mL
1 tsp	GF baking powder	5 mL
2 tsp	baking soda	10 mL
½ tsp	salt	2 mL
1½ tsp	ground cinnamon	7 mL
½ tsp	ground nutmeg	2 mL
3	eggs	3
1¼ cups	granulated sugar	300 mL
¾ cup	GF sour cream	175 mL
1 cup	crushed pineapple, including juice	250 mL
2 cups	shredded carrots	500 mL
¾ cup	chopped walnuts	175 mL

1. In a large bowl, sift together brown rice flour, soy flour, potato starch, tapioca starch, xanthan gum, baking powder, baking soda, salt, cinnamon and nutmeg. Resift and set aside.

2. In a separate bowl, using an electric mixer, beat eggs, sugar, sour cream and pineapple until well blended. Gradually beat in dry ingredients. Stir in carrots and walnuts.

3. Spoon into prepared pan. Spread to edges and smooth top with a moist rubber spatula. Let stand for 30 minutes.

4. Bake in preheated oven for 50 to 60 minutes or until a cake tester inserted in the center comes out clean. Let cool in the pan on a rack for 10 minutes. Remove from pan and let cool completely on rack.

Rhubarb Crumb Cake

SERVES 9 TO 12

Looking for more ways to use the first harvest of the season? All summer long, Susan, one of our taste testers, kept requesting more of this one.

TIPS

This cake stays moist for lunch or an afternoon snack.

∾

Once frozen, this cake tends to crumble more easily. Freeze it in individual servings, wrapped airtight, then microwave for just a few seconds to warm them up.

VARIATION

Add ¾ cup (175 mL) finely chopped pecans to the topping and ½ cup (125 mL) coarsely chopped pecans to the cake batter.

Preheat oven to 350°F (180°C)
8-inch (2 L) square pan, lightly greased

¼ cup	packed brown sugar	50 mL
1 tbsp	orange zest	15 mL
½ tsp	ground cinnamon	2 mL
¾ cup	brown rice flour	175 mL
¾ cup	sorghum flour	175 mL
⅓ cup	tapioca starch	75 mL
¾ cup	granulated sugar	175 mL
¾ tsp	xanthan gum	4 mL
2 tsp	GF baking powder	10 mL
½ tsp	baking soda	2 mL
½ tsp	salt	2 mL
2	eggs	2
⅓ cup	vegetable oil	75 mL
1 tsp	vanilla extract	5 mL
1 tsp	orange zest	5 mL
1 cup	freshly squeezed orange juice	250 mL
2 cups	chopped rhubarb	500 mL

1. In a small bowl, combine brown sugar, orange zest and cinnamon. Set aside for topping.

2. In a large bowl or plastic bag, sift brown rice flour, sorghum flour, tapioca starch, sugar, xanthan gum, baking powder, baking soda and salt. Resift and set aside.

3. In a separate large bowl, using an electric mixer, beat eggs, oil, vanilla extract, orange zest and orange juice until combined. With mixer on low, slowly add dry ingredients and mix just until smooth. Fold in rhubarb and spoon into prepared pan. Spread to edges and smooth top with a moist rubber spatula. Sprinkle with topping. Let stand for 30 minutes.

4. Bake in preheated oven for 50 to 60 minutes or until a cake tester inserted in the center comes out clean. Let cool completely in the pan on a rack.

Raspberry-Filled Jelly Roll

SERVES 8 TO 10

A cookbook would not be complete without a jelly roll recipe. Heather has fond memories of this raspberry-filled treat being prepared by her grandmother every Saturday for lunch.

TIPS

For better volume, while beating egg whites, make sure the bowl and beaters are completely free of grease and egg yolk. Wash these, right before using them.

∽

Wrap filled or unfilled jelly roll airtight and freeze for up to 1 month.

Preheat oven to 400°F (200°C)
15-by 10-inch (40 by 25 cm) jelly roll pan, lightly greased, then lined with parchment or waxed paper

⅓ cup	brown rice flour	75 mL
⅓ cup	soy flour	75 mL
2 tbsp	tapioca starch	25 mL
1 tsp	xanthan gum	5 mL
¾ tsp	GF baking powder	4 mL
¼ tsp	salt	1 mL
4	egg yolks	4
4	egg whites, warmed to room temperature (see Techniques Glossary, page 178)	4
¾ cup	granulated sugar	175 mL
½ tsp	lemon flavoring	2 mL
	GF confectioner's (icing) sugar	
1 cup	raspberry jam	250 mL

1. In a bowl, sift together brown rice flour, soy flour, tapioca starch, xanthan gum, baking powder and salt. Resift and set aside.

2. In a small bowl, using an electric mixer, beat egg yolks until thick and lemon colored, approximately 5 minutes. Set aside.

Substitute a flavored
whipped cream, grape
jelly, peach, apricot
or strawberry jam
for the jam.

3. In a separate large bowl, using an electric mixer beat egg whites until stiff. Gradually add sugar. Continue beating until mixture is very stiff and glossy but not dry.

4. Fold beaten yolks into beaten whites. Add lemon flavoring. Fold in dry ingredients. Spoon into prepared pan. Carefully spread to the edges with a moist rubber spatula. Let stand for 30 minutes. Bake in preheated oven for 10 to 12 minutes or until the top springs back when lightly touched.

5. Dust lightly with confectioner's sugar. Turn out onto a clean tea towel. Carefully remove paper. Starting at the short side, immediately roll up in the tea towel. Let cool on a rack for 15 minutes.

6. Unroll cake and spread with raspberry jam. Roll up again and place, seam-side down, on serving platter. Cover and refrigerate for 30 to 60 minutes before serving.

Applesauce-Date Snacking Cake

SERVES 6 TO 8

No need to feel guilty! You would never guess this deliciously moist cake is low in fat, too! Serve with clementines in season or add a sweet touch of Orange Glaze (see recipe, page 155).

TIP

When purchasing chopped dates, check for wheat starch in the coating.

VARIATIONS

For a more intense flavor, substitute brown rice flour for the sorghum.

∽

Substitute dried figs or prunes for dates.

Preheat oven to 350°F (180°C)
8-inch (2 L) square pan, lightly greased

⅔ cup	whole bean flour	150 mL
⅔ cup	sorghum flour	150 mL
¼ cup	tapioca starch	50 mL
1 tsp	xanthan gum	5 mL
½ tsp	GF baking powder	2 mL
½ tsp	baking soda	2 mL
⅛ tsp	salt	0.5 mL
1 tsp	unsweetened cocoa powder	5 mL
1 tsp	ground cinnamon	5 mL
¼ tsp	ground nutmeg	1 mL
⅛ tsp	ground cloves	0.5 mL
¼ cup	butter or shortening, softened	50 mL
½ cup	packed brown sugar	125 mL
1	egg	1
1 tsp	vanilla extract	5 mL
1 cup	unsweetened applesauce	250 mL
¾ cup	chopped dates	175 mL

1. In a large bowl, sift together whole bean flour, sorghum flour, tapioca starch, xanthan gum, baking powder, baking soda, salt, cocoa, cinnamon, nutmeg and cloves. Resift and set aside.

2. In a separate bowl, using an electric mixer, cream butter and brown sugar. Add egg and vanilla extract. Beat until light and fluffy.

3. Stir in dry ingredients, alternately with applesauce, to butter-sugar mixture, making three additions of dry ingredients and two of applesauce. Stir just until combined after each addition. Stir in dates. Spoon batter into prepared pan. Spread to edges and smooth top with a moist rubber spatula. Let stand for 30 minutes.

4. Bake in preheated oven for 25 to 30 minutes or until a cake tester inserted in the center comes out clean. Let cake cool in the pan on a rack for 10 minutes. Remove from pan and let cool completely on a rack.

Gingered Pumpkin Snacking Cake

It's perfect for a
Halloween party —
but serve this moist
spice cake year round.
It makes an excellent
snack to carry in
lunches or for a
mid-morning break.

TIPS

Fresh gingerroot
has too strong a flavor
to substitute for
the candied or
crystallized ginger.

❧

Be sure to buy pumpkin
purée, not pumpkin pie
filling, which is too
sweet and contains too
much moisture for this
snacking cake.

Preheat oven to 350°F (180°C)
13-by 9-inch (3 L) baking pan, lightly greased

1 cup	sorghum flour	250 mL
¾ cup	whole bean flour	175 mL
¼ cup	potato starch	50 mL
¼ cup	tapioca starch	50 mL
2 tsp	xanthan gum	10 mL
1½ tsp	GF baking powder	7 mL
¾ tsp	baking soda	4 mL
½ tsp	salt	2 mL
1 tsp	ground cinnamon	5 mL
½ tsp	ground allspice	2 mL
½ tsp	ground ginger	2 mL
½ tsp	ground nutmeg	2 mL
½ cup	butter or shortening, softened	125 mL
1 cup	packed brown sugar	250 mL
¼ cup	frozen orange juice concentrate, thawed	50 mL
2	eggs	2
1 tsp	vanilla extract	5 mL
1 cup	canned pumpkin purée (not pie filling)	250 mL
½ cup	chopped pecans	125 mL
⅓ cup	chopped candied or crystallized ginger	75 mL

For a stronger pumpkin flavor, omit the candied or crystallized ginger.

∾

To dress up this snacking cake, drizzle it with double the Orange Glaze (see recipe, page 155).

1. In a large bowl, sift together sorghum flour, whole bean flour, potato starch, tapioca starch, xanthan gum, baking powder, baking soda, salt, cinnamon, allspice, ginger and nutmeg. Resift and set aside.

2. In a separate bowl, using an electric mixer, cream butter and brown sugar. Add orange juice, eggs, vanilla extract and pumpkin purée and beat well. Gradually beat in dry ingredients, mixing just until smooth, about 2 minutes. Stir in pecans and candied ginger. Spoon into prepared pan. Spread to edges and smooth top with a moist rubber spatula. Let stand for 30 minutes.

3. Bake in preheated oven for 25 to 35 minutes or until a cake tester inserted in the center comes out clean. Let cool in the pan on a rack for 10 minutes. Remove from the pan and let cool completely on a rack.

Sticky Bun Snacking Cake

SERVES 6 TO 8

Traditional sticky buns require a lot of patience as you wait for the dough to rise. This version is ready in no time!

TIPS

For easier pouring, warm the corn syrup in the microwave for 50 seconds on High.

∾

Line the bottom of the lightly greased pan with waxed or parchment paper.

VARIATION

Substitute walnuts or raisins for pecans in the topping.

Preheat oven to 350°F (180°C)
9-inch (2.5 L) square pan, lightly greased

TOPPING

1 cup	coarsely chopped pecans	250 mL
1 cup	halved red and green glacé cherries	250 mL
½ cup	packed brown sugar	125 mL
2 tsp	ground cinnamon	10 mL
¼ cup	melted butter	50 mL

CAKE

1¼ cups	white rice flour	300 mL
½ cup	potato starch	125 mL
¼ cup	tapioca starch	50 mL
½ cup	granulated sugar	125 mL
1½ tsp	xanthan gum	7 mL
1 tsp	GF baking powder	5 mL
1 tsp	baking soda	5 mL
¼ tsp	salt	1 mL
1¼ cups	plain yogurt	300 mL
1 tsp	cider vinegar	5 mL
¼ cup	vegetable oil	50 mL
2	eggs	2
½ cup	corn syrup, warmed (see Tip, left)	125 mL

1. *Topping:* In a small bowl, combine pecans, glacé cherries, brown sugar and cinnamon. Add melted butter and mix well. Spread into prepared pan.

2. *Cake:* In a large bowl, stir together white rice flour, potato starch, tapioca starch, sugar, xanthan gum, baking powder, baking soda and salt. Resift and set aside.

3. In a separate bowl, using an electric mixer or whisk, beat yogurt, vinegar, oil and eggs until combined. Pour mixture over dry ingredients and stir just until combined. Spoon over topping in prepared pan. Spread to edges and smooth top with a moist rubber spatula. Let stand for 30 minutes.

4. Bake in preheated oven for 30 to 35 minutes or until a cake tester inserted in the center comes out clean. Immediately turn upside down on a serving platter and remove pan. Drizzle cake with warm corn syrup. Serve warm.

Cranberry-Banana Cupcakes

MAKES 12 CUPCAKES

This easy-to-carry cupcake can be put in a lunch bag, still frozen. It will help keep your sandwich cold.

TIPS

Mash and freeze ripe bananas so they are ready when you need them. Thaw and bring to room temperature before using.

❧

Fill muffin cups almost level with the top.

VARIATIONS

Substitute fresh or dried blueberries, dried cherries or golden raisins for the cranberries.

❧

For a traditional banana cake, spoon batter into a lightly greased 9-inch (2.5 L) square baking pan and bake for 35 minutes or until a cake tester inserted in the center comes out clean.

Preheat oven to 350°F (180°C)
Muffin tins, lightly greased

¾ cup	sorghum flour	175 mL
¾ cup	soy flour	175 mL
¼ cup	potato starch	50 mL
¼ cup	tapioca starch	50 mL
2 tsp	xanthan gum	10 mL
1 tsp	GF baking powder	5 mL
¾ tsp	baking soda	4 mL
½ tsp	salt	2 mL
¼ cup	vegetable oil	50 mL
2	eggs	2
1 cup	packed brown sugar	250 mL
1 tsp	vanilla extract	5 mL
1 cup	mashed banana, about 2 to 3 (see Tips, left)	250 mL
½ cup	plain yogurt	125 mL
1 cup	dried cranberries	250 mL

1. In a large bowl, sift together sorghum flour, soy flour, potato starch, tapioca starch, xanthan gum, baking powder, baking soda and salt. Resift and set aside.

2. In a separate bowl, using an electric mixer, beat together oil and eggs. While beating, add brown sugar, vanilla extract, bananas and yogurt. Beat until well blended. Gradually beat in dry ingredients, mixing just until smooth, about 2 minutes. Stir in cranberries. Spoon into each cup of prepared muffin tins. Let stand for 30 minutes.

3. Bake in preheated oven for 20 to 25 minutes or until a cake tester inserted in the center comes out clean. Let cool in the pan on a rack for 5 minutes. Remove from the pan and let cool completely on a rack.

Orange Glaze

MAKES ⅓ CUP (75 ML)

½ cup	GF sifted confectioner's (icing) sugar	125 mL
2 tsp	frozen orange juice concentrate, thawed	10 mL

Don't want the extra calories in a frosting? Drizzle just enough glaze for a tangy sweet orange taste. It complements the flavor of the Applesauce-Date Snacking Cake (see recipe, page 148).

1. In a small bowl, stir together confectioner's sugar and orange juice concentrate. Drizzle over cooled cake.

TIP

Sift confectioner's sugar to remove lumps before adding the orange juice.

Chocolate Glaze

MAKES 1 CUP (250 ML)

½ cup	unsweetened cocoa powder	125 mL
2 tbsp	granulated sugar	25 mL
2 tbsp	cornstarch	25 mL
⅓ cup	milk	75 mL
¼ cup	corn syrup	50 mL
1 tsp	vanilla extract	5 mL

Great for Chocolate Fudge Cake, Angel Food Cake or White Cake (see recipes, pages 140, 141 and 142).

1. In a small saucepan, sift together cocoa, sugar and cornstarch. Whisk in milk, corn syrup and vanilla extract. Bring to a boil over medium heat, stirring constantly, until glaze boils. Boil for 1 to 2 minutes until thickened and glossy. Cool 5 minutes. Drizzle over cooled cake.

TIP

To eliminate lumps, sift together cocoa, sugar and cornstarch before adding the liquids.

VARIATION

Use as a chocolate syrup to make chocolate milk.

Orange Frosting

MAKES 2⅓ CUPS
(575 ML)

We love a chocolate-orange flavor combination. This is great with our Chocolate Fudge Cake (see recipe, page 140), but it suits any kind of cake, from chocolate to white to angel food.

TIP

Check for gluten-free confectioner's (icing) sugar. In Canada, it may contain up to 5% starch, which could be from wheat.

½ cup	shortening or butter, softened	125 mL
4 cups	GF sifted confectioner's (icing) sugar (see Tip, left)	1 L
2 tbsp	orange zest	25 mL
¼ cup	freshly squeezed orange juice	50 mL
2 tbsp	orange liqueur	25 mL

1. In a bowl, using an electric mixer, beat shortening, confectioner's sugar, orange zest, juice and liqueur until smooth and creamy. Spread over cooled cake.

Cream Cheese Frosting

MAKES ENOUGH TO FROST 1 CAKE

The only acceptable finish for Pineapple-Carrot Cake (see recipe, page 144) or any carrot cake is Cream Cheese Frosting. Also great over Gingered Pumpkin Snacking Cake (see recipe, page 150).

1	package (8 oz/250 g) cream cheese, at room temperature	1
½ cup	butter, softened	125 mL
2 cups	GF sifted confectioner's (icing) sugar	500 mL
1 tsp	vanilla extract	5 mL

1. In a bowl, using an electric mixer, beat cream cheese and butter until light and fluffy. Beat in confectioner's sugar and vanilla extract. Spread over cooled cake.

Sweet Treats

*If you're packing a lunch or visiting a friend,
take along a few treats to nibble when
you crave a little sweetness.*

~ Cookie and Bar Tips ~

- Granulated sugar generally results in crisper cookies than either brown sugar or honey. Equal amounts may be substituted one for the other or a combination of sugars may be used. Experiment to see what you prefer.

- Using butter in a cookie usually causes the dough to spread more, giving a flatter, crisper cookie than when made with shortening. You can substitute or use part of each in a recipe to give the texture you want.

- Bake a test cookie to check the accuracy of your oven's temperature setting. You may need to increase or reduce the temperature slightly or adjust the baking time. This is a good time to check the consistency of the dough. Add 1 to 2 tbsp (15 to 25 mL) sweet rice flour if the dough is too soft, causing the cookie to spread out more than you might like.

- When making cookies, make dough for about 4 to 6 dozen. Bake 1 or 2 dozen and form the remaining dough into logs. Each log should have enough dough to make 1 or 2 dozen cookies. Freeze these logs and, when making more cookies, there is no need to thaw the dough completely. Let a log thaw just enough to be able to slice it in $1/2$-inch (1 cm) circles. Baking a small amount at one time ensures you have fresh cookies without the work of making the dough each time. Dough can be frozen for up to 1 month.

- If the dough is a bit stickier than normal, flour the board and/or your fingertips with sweet rice flour. Use rice flour if it's of normal consistency.

- Shiny baking sheets produce soft-bottomed cookies, while darker pans result in crisper cookies.

- When baked, remove cookies from the baking sheet and place, without overlapping, on a wire rack, to cool completely.

- Store soft cookies in an airtight container so they stay soft and moist. Crisp cookies should be lightly wrapped in a covered, but not airtight container.

- Freeze cookies and bars between sheets of waxed paper for up to 6 months.

Apricot Coconut Balls

MAKES 4 DOZEN COOKIES

Not too sweet, not too wet, not too dry — but just right for a portable snack at any time of the year. Use these treats like an energy bar for your favorite athlete or on a tray of gluten-free holiday goodies.

TIPS

If the fruit mixture is not processed finely enough, the cookie is harder to form and falls apart easily.

~

Make ahead and store in an airtight container for up to 1 month.

VARIATIONS

Any dried fruit combination works well. Keep the total amount of fruit to 2½ cups (625 mL).

~

Substitute orange juice for brandy.

Baking sheets, lined with waxed paper

1 cup	chopped dried apricots	250 mL
½ cup	chopped dried figs	125 mL
½ cup	chopped dried prunes	125 mL
½ cup	chopped dried apples	125 mL
3 tbsp	flavored brandy	45 mL
1 tbsp	orange zest	15 mL
1¼ cups	sweetened desiccated coconut, divided	300 mL
¾ cup	chopped nuts, such as walnuts	175 mL

1. In a glass pie plate, combine apricots, figs, prunes, apples, brandy and orange zest. Cover and let stand for at least 1 hour or overnight.

2. In a food processor or blender, pulse dried fruit mixture until finely chopped. Mix in ¾ cup (175 mL) coconut and nuts. Pulse until nuts are chopped and mixture holds together easily.

3. Shape into ¾-inch (2 cm) balls. Roll in remaining ½ cup (125 mL) coconut. Let stand on prepared pans for 8 hours or overnight.

Chocolate Chip Cookies

MAKES 6 ½ DOZEN COOKIES

> *No point trying to freeze these — the minute anyone knows they are in the house, the cookies disappear.*

TIP

For crisper cookies, replace shortening with butter or margarine and substitute half the brown sugar with granulated sugar.

VARIATIONS

Substitute white chocolate chips and macadamia nuts for mini-chocolate chips and walnuts.

∾

To bake a dozen cookies at a time or to turn these into slice-and-bake cookies, form the dough into 1-inch (2.5 cm) logs 6 inches (15 cm) in length, and freeze for up to 1 month. To bake, thaw slightly and cut into ½-inch (1 cm) slices. Bake 10 to 12 minutes.

Preheat oven to 350°F (180°C)
Baking sheets, lightly greased

1 cup	sorghum flour	250 mL
⅔ cup	whole bean flour	150 mL
½ cup	tapioca starch	125 mL
1 tsp	baking soda	5 mL
1 tsp	xanthan gum	5 mL
½ tsp	salt	2 mL
1 cup	shortening, softened	250 mL
1⅓ cups	packed brown sugar	325 mL
2	eggs	2
1 tsp	vanilla extract	5 mL
2 cups	mini-chocolate chips	500 mL
1 cup	chopped walnuts	250 mL

1. In a bowl or plastic bag, combine sorghum flour, whole bean flour, tapioca starch, baking soda, xanthan gum and salt. Mix well and set aside.

2. In a separate bowl, using an electric mixer, cream shortening and brown sugar. Add eggs and vanilla extract and beat until light and fluffy. Slowly beat in the dry ingredients until combined. Stir in chocolate chips and walnuts. Drop dough by level teaspoonfuls (15 mL), 1½ inches (4 cm) apart on prepared baking sheets. Let stand for 30 minutes. Bake in preheated oven for 8 to 10 minutes or until set. Remove from baking sheets to a cooling rack immediately.

Peachy Plum Hazelnut Galette (page 133)

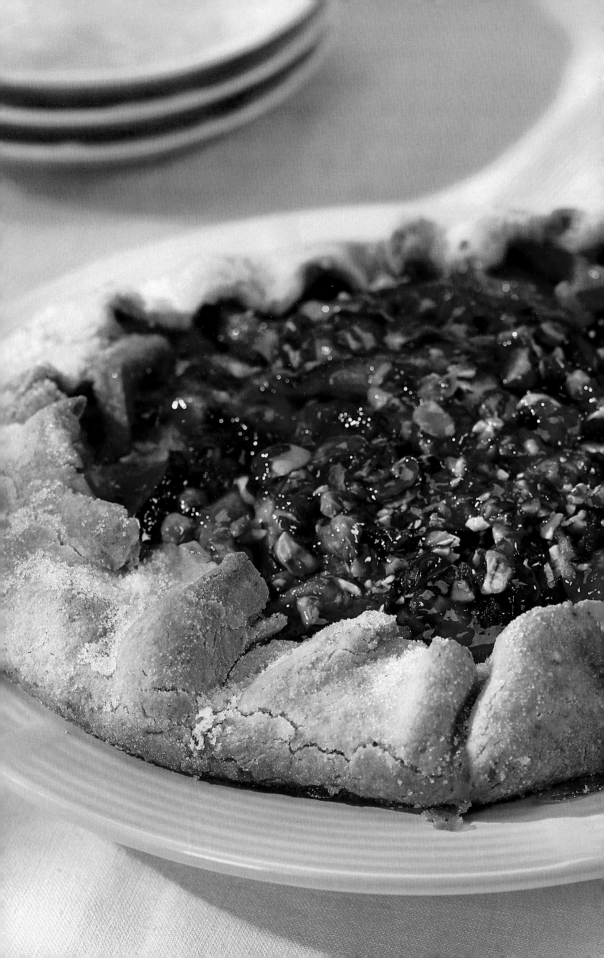

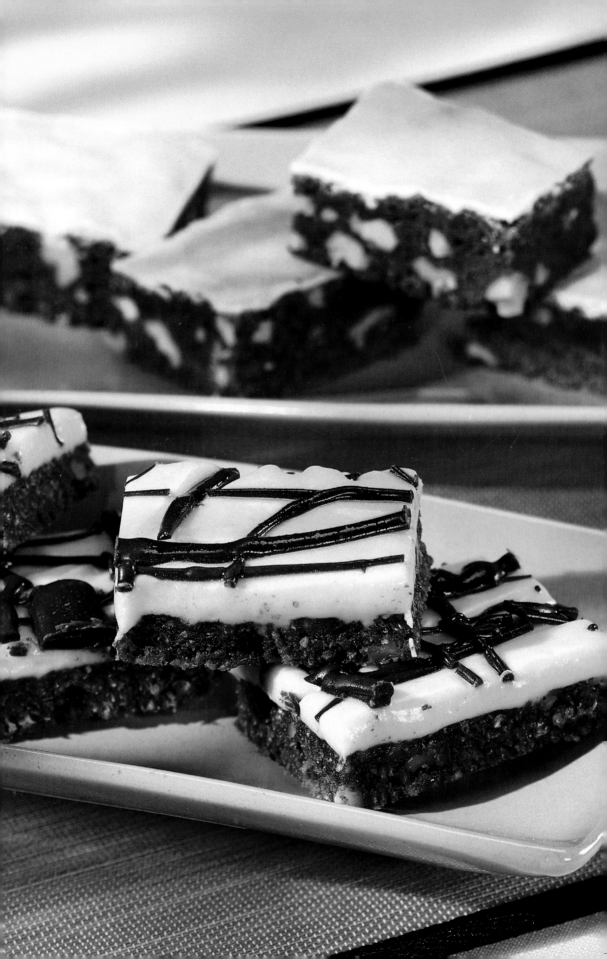

Cranberry Drops

MAKES 3 DOZEN COOKIES

These cookies are a lunchbox favorite! Hermit-like in color and soft in texture, each bite has the tang of fresh cranberries.

TIPS

Cool the baking sheet before re-using it to prevent the dough from spreading too much.

∽

Leave cranberries in the freezer until just before adding to the dough. This helps to prevent them from "bleeding" into the cookies.

∽

Freeze raw dough, formed into cookies, for approximately 1 hour then place them in an airtight freezer bag. Freeze for up to 1 month. Bake from frozen for 15 to 18 minutes.

VARIATION

Substitute fresh or frozen blueberries for the cranberries.

Fudgy Brownies (page 168) and Nanaimo Bars (page 170)

Preheat oven to 350°F (180°C)
Baking sheets, lightly greased

1 cup	brown rice flour	250 mL
1/3 cup	yellow pea flour or whole bean flour (see Tips, page 167)	75 mL
2 tbsp	tapioca starch	25 mL
1/2 tsp	baking soda	2 mL
1 tsp	xanthan gum	5 mL
1/4 tsp	salt	1 mL
1/4 cup	shortening or butter, softened	50 mL
3/4 cup	packed brown sugar	175 mL
1	egg	1
3 tbsp	milk	45 mL
1/2 tsp	vanilla extract	2 mL
3/4 cup	cranberries, fresh or frozen	175 mL
1/2 cup	chopped walnuts	125 mL

1. In a bowl, sift brown rice flour, yellow pea flour, tapioca starch, baking soda, xanthan gum and salt. Mix well and set aside.

2. In a separate bowl, using an electric mixer, cream shortening and brown sugar. Add egg, milk and vanilla extract. Beat until light and fluffy. Slowly beat in the dry ingredients until combined. Stir in cranberries and walnuts. Drop dough by rounded tablespoonfuls (15 mL), 2 inches (5 cm) apart on prepared baking sheets. Let stand for 30 minutes. Bake in preheated oven for 12 to 15 minutes or until set. Transfer to a cooling rack immediately.

Mini-Thumbprints

MAKES 4 TO 4½ DOZEN COOKIES

Preheat oven to 350°F (180°C)
Baking sheets, lightly greased

> *Thumbprint cookies, thimble cookies or Swedish tea rings — by whatever name you know them — are so rich that the bite-size morsels melt in your mouth. So tender and delicate, they are not meant to carry for lunch.*

TIPS
To prevent cookies from crumbling, leave them on the baking sheet for 2 to 3 minutes after you take them from the oven. Then remove them carefully. The one that breaks is your reward for baking.

∾

Nuts must be very finely chopped to generously coat the cookies.

VARIATIONS
Substitute apricot, raspberry or black currant jam or jelly for the grape.

∾

Instead of jam or jelly, fill the indent with melted chocolate.

COOKIE

1 cup	rice flour	250 mL
⅔ cup	cornstarch	150 mL
⅔ cup	GF confectioner's (icing) sugar	150 mL
⅓ cup	potato starch	75 mL
1 tsp	xanthan gum	5 mL
¾ cup	butter, softened	175 mL
1	egg yolk	1

COATING

2	egg whites, lightly beaten	2
1 tbsp	water	15 mL
1½ cups	finely chopped walnuts (see Tips, left)	375 mL
½ cup	grape jelly	125 mL

1. *Cookie:* In a bowl or plastic bag, combine rice flour, cornstarch, confectioner's sugar, potato starch and xanthan gum. Mix well and set aside.

2. In a separate bowl, using an electric mixer, beat butter and egg yolk until light and fluffy. Slowly beat in the dry ingredients until combined. With a rubber spatula, scrape the bottom and sides of bowl. Gather the dough into a large ball, kneading in any remaining dry ingredients. Form into ½-inch (1 cm) balls.

3. *Coating:* In a small bowl, combine egg whites and water.

4. Roll cookies in egg white mixture and then in nuts. Place 1 inch (2.5 cm) apart on prepared baking sheets. Using the end of the handle of a wooden spoon, make an indent in the center of each. Bake in preheated oven for 8 minutes then remove from the oven, deepen indent and bake for an additional 6 to 8 minutes or until golden. Let stand for 2 to 3 minutes. Carefully transfer to a cooling rack immediately. Let cool slightly and fill the indent with jelly.

Peanut Butter Cookies

MAKES 3 DOZEN COOKIES

Everybody's absolute favorite cookie! These are just perfect to share with friends of all ages. No need to be separate from the crowd!

TIP

Roll dough into logs 1½ inches (4 cm) in diameter. Wrap airtight and refrigerate for 1 week or freeze for up to 1 month to bake later. Thaw slightly and bake for 10 to 12 minutes. You decide the length of the log, depending on the number of cookies you want to bake. Cut partially thawed logs into ½-inch (1 cm) slices to bake.

VARIATIONS

Substitute chunky peanut butter for smooth and add ½ cup (125 mL) chopped peanuts.

∾

For a chewy peanut butter cookie, add an extra egg.

Preheat oven to 350°F (180°C)
Baking sheets, ungreased

1 cup	soy flour	250 mL
½ cup	packed brown sugar	125 mL
½ cup	granulated sugar	125 mL
⅓ cup	cornstarch	75 mL
½ tsp	baking soda	2 mL
½ tsp	xanthan gum	2 mL
¼ tsp	salt	1 mL
½ cup	butter, softened	125 mL
½ cup	smooth peanut butter	125 mL
1	egg	1
½ tsp	vanilla extract	2 mL
	Sweet rice flour (optional)	

1. In a bowl or plastic bag, combine soy flour, brown sugar, granulated sugar, cornstarch, baking soda, xanthan gum and salt. Mix well and set aside.

2. In a separate bowl, using an electric mixer, cream butter and peanut butter. Add egg and vanilla. Beat until light and fluffy. Slowly stir in the dry ingredients until combined. With a rubber spatula, scrape the bottom and sides of bowl.

3. Gather the dough into a large ball, kneading in any remaining dry ingredients. Roll into 1-inch (2.5 cm) balls. Place 1½ inches (4 cm) apart on the baking sheets. Flatten slightly with a fork dipped into sweet rice flour, if necessary, to prevent sticking. Bake in preheated oven for 10 to 15 minutes or until set. Transfer to a cooling rack immediately.

Sue's Shortbread

MAKES 2½ DOZEN
COOKIES

*Sue Jennett, of
Kingston, Ontario,
diagnosed with celiac
disease years ago, gave
us her recipe for
shortbread to share
with you.*

TIP

As the dough is soft,
handle gently when
rolling into balls and try
not to add extra flour.

VARIATION

Prick with a fork, bake
and then sprinkle the
tops with a little extra
fine sugar while
still warm.

Preheat oven to 300°F (150°C)
Baking sheets, ungreased

⅔ cup	rice flour	150 mL
½ cup	cornstarch	125 mL
½ cup	GF sifted confectioner's (icing) sugar	125 mL
¼ cup	potato starch	50 mL
2 tbsp	tapioca starch	25 mL
¾ cup	butter, softened	175 mL
	Sweet rice flour (optional)	

1. In a bowl or plastic bag, combine rice flour, cornstarch, confectioner's sugar, potato starch and tapioca starch. Mix well and set aside.

2. In a separate bowl, using an electric mixer, cream butter. Slowly beat in the dry ingredients until combined. With a rubber spatula, scrape the bottom and sides of bowl.

3. Gather the dough into a large ball, kneading in any remaining dry ingredients. Roll into 1-inch (2.5 cm) balls. Place 1 inch (2.5 cm) apart on baking sheets. If desired, flatten with fork dipped into sweet rice flour. Bake in preheated oven for 15 to 25 minutes or until set but not browned. Transfer to a cooling rack immediately.

Butter Tart Bars

MAKES 3 DOZEN BARS

> *A most important Canadian treat, these are a much sought-after addition to any dessert tray. They disappear first.*

TIP
The shortbread base tends to crumble if cut while the bars are still warm. Refrigerated overnight, the bars cut more easily.

VARIATIONS
Omit the nuts and add an equal amount of butterscotch or peanut butter chips or unsweetened coconut.

∽

Substitute an equal amount of egg replacer for the xanthan gum. Add ¼ tsp (1 mL) salt.

Preheat oven to 350°F (180°C)
9-inch (2.5 L) square pan, ungreased

BASE

1 cup	rice flour	250 mL
⅓ cup	tapioca starch	75 mL
⅓ cup	packed brown sugar	75 mL
2 tbsp	potato starch	25 mL
1 tsp	xanthan gum	5 mL
½ cup	butter, softened	125 mL

TOPPING

2 tbsp	cornstarch	25 mL
½ tsp	GF baking powder	2 mL
¼ tsp	salt	1 mL
2	eggs	2
¾ cup	corn syrup	175 mL
1 cup	raisins	250 mL
½ cup	chopped walnuts	125 mL

1. *Base:* In a bowl or plastic bag, combine rice flour, tapioca starch, brown sugar, potato starch and xanthan gum. Mix well and set aside.

2. In a separate bowl, using an electric mixer, cream butter. Slowly beat in the dry ingredients until combined. With a rubber spatula, scrape the bottom and sides of bowl. Press into the bottom of pan. Bake in preheated oven for 10 minutes or until set but not browned. Meanwhile, prepare Topping.

3. *Topping:* In a small bowl, combine cornstarch, baking powder and salt. Set aside.

4. In a separate bowl, using an electric mixer, beat eggs until light and fluffy. Add corn syrup while mixing. With the mixer on low, slowly add dry ingredients and mix just until smooth. Do not over mix. Fold in raisins and walnuts and pour over the hot base. Bake in preheated oven for 25 to 35 minutes or until the center is almost firm. Refrigerate overnight before cutting into squares.

Cinnamon Crisps

MAKES 3 DOZEN BARS

> *Give cinnamon lovers these sweet, crunchy snacks any time!*

TIPS
The dough is very stiff but still rolls out easily.

∼

Cut bars while warm as they become too crisp to cut when they are cool.

VARIATION
Make three kinds of cookies at the same time. Divide dough into thirds. Sprinkle one portion with chopped pecans. Then choose chocolate, butterscotch, peanut butter, raspberry or cinnamon chips for the other two portions.

Preheat 300°F (150°C)
15-by 10-inch (40 by 25 cm) jelly roll pan, greased

1²/₃ cups	soy flour	400 mL
¹/₃ cup	tapioca starch	75 mL
¹/₂ tsp	baking soda	2 mL
1 tsp	xanthan gum	5 mL
¹/₄ tsp	salt	1 mL
1 tbsp	ground cinnamon	15 mL
1 cup	butter, softened	250 mL
¹/₂ cup	packed brown sugar	125 mL
¹/₂ cup	granulated sugar	125 mL
1	egg, separated	1
1¹/₂ cups	chopped pecans	375 mL

1. In a bowl or plastic bag, combine soy flour, tapioca starch, baking soda, xanthan gum, salt and cinnamon. Mix well and set aside.

2. In a separate bowl, using an electric mixer, cream butter, brown sugar, granulated sugar and egg yolk until light and fluffy. Slowly beat in the dry ingredients until combined.

3. Form the dough into a large disk and place in the prepared pan. Cover with waxed paper. With a rolling pin, roll out the dough to fit the pan. Carefully remove the waxed paper.

4. In a small bowl, beat egg white with a fork just until foamy. Brush on top of dough. Sprinkle with pecans and press them in lightly. Let stand for 30 minutes. Bake in preheated oven for 35 to 45 minutes or until set. Immediately cut into bars. Let cool in the pan.

Crunchy Blondies

MAKES 1½ DOZEN BLONDIES

Full of toffee bits and white chocolate chips, these thin, chewy blond brownies are quick and easy to make.

TIPS

We like to sift the dry ingredients when using yellow pea flour because it lumps easily.

❧

Yellow pea flour gives baked products a warm golden color.

VARIATION

Double the toffee bits and eliminate the white chocolate chips or double the white chocolate chips and eliminate the toffee bits.

Preheat oven to 350°F (180°C)
13-by 9-inch (3 L) baking pan, lightly greased

¾ cup	brown rice flour	175 mL
½ cup	yellow pea flour or whole bean flour (see Tips, left)	125 mL
¼ cup	tapioca starch	50 mL
2 tsp	GF baking powder	10 mL
2 tsp	xanthan gum	10 mL
¼ tsp	salt	1 mL
½ cup	butter, softened	125 mL
¾ cup	granulated sugar	175 mL
⅓ cup	packed brown sugar	75 mL
2	eggs	2
1 tsp	vanilla extract	5 mL
½ cup	toffee bits	125 mL
½ cup	white chocolate chips	125 mL

1. In a large bowl, sift together brown rice flour, yellow pea flour, tapioca starch, baking powder, xanthan gum and salt. Resift and set aside.

2. In a separate bowl, using an electric mixer, cream butter, granulated sugar and brown sugar. Add eggs and vanilla extract. Beat until light and fluffy. Gradually beat in dry ingredients, mixing just until smooth. Stir in toffee bits and white chocolate chips. Spoon into prepared pan, spread to edges and smooth top with a moist rubber spatula. Let stand for 30 minutes.

3. Bake in preheated oven for 35 to 45 minutes or until a wooden skewer inserted in the center comes out clean. Transfer to cooling rack and let cool completely. Cut into bars.

Fudgy Brownies

MAKES 16 BROWNIES

> *Doubly delicious, these moist, fudgy brownies appeal to the eye as well as the taste of every chocoholic!*

TIP

One individually wrapped square of baking chocolate is 1 oz (30 g). For further instructions on melting chocolate, see Chocolate, page 178.

VARIATIONS

Substitute an equal amount of whole bean flour for yellow pea.

❦

Keep extra brownies in the freezer. Crumb them and use as a base for cheesecake or cube them for a chocolate trifle.

Preheat oven to 350°F (180°C)
8-inch (2 L) square pan, lightly greased

⅓ cup	yellow pea flour	75 mL
2 tbsp	potato starch	25 mL
1 cup	packed brown sugar	250 mL
½ tsp	GF baking powder	2 mL
½ tsp	xanthan gum	2 mL
⅛ tsp	salt	0.5 mL
½ cup	chopped walnuts	125 mL
½ cup	shortening	125 mL
2 oz	unsweetened chocolate	60 g
½ tsp	vanilla extract	2 mL
2	eggs	2

GLAZE (OPTIONAL)

2 tsp	shortening	10 mL
2 oz	white chocolate	60 g

1. In a large bowl or plastic bag, combine yellow pea flour, potato starch, brown sugar, baking powder, xanthan gum, salt and walnuts. Mix well and set aside.

2. In a large bowl, microwave shortening and chocolate on Medium for 3 minutes or until partially melted in a saucepan over hot water. Stir until melted. Add eggs, one at a time, blending after each. Stir in vanilla extract. Slowly add the dry ingredients, stirring until combined. Spread evenly in prepared pan. Let stand for 30 minutes. Bake in a preheated oven for 20 to 25 minutes or until a cake tester inserted in the center still has a little moist crumb adhering to it. Transfer to a rack to cool completely. Let cool for 15 minutes on rack. Meanwhile, prepare glaze, if desired.

3. *Glaze:* In a small bowl, over hot water, partially melt the shortening and chocolate. Remove from heat and continue stirring until completely melted. Spread on warm brownies. Cool completely before cutting into squares.

Hazelnut Apricot Bars

MAKES 2 DOZEN BARS

> *Imagine the flavors of sweet apricot and creamy white chocolate combined with crunchy hazelnuts — just don't count the calories!*

TIPS

For further instructions on melting chocolate, see Chocolate, page 178.

⁓

If hazelnut flour is not readily available in your area, see Nut Flour, page 180, for instructions to make your own.

VARIATION

Substitute an equal amount of egg replacer for the xanthan gum. Add ¼ tsp (1 mL) salt.

Preheat oven to 325°F (160°C)

9-inch (2.5 L) square pan, lightly greased

BASE

¾ cup	rice flour	175 mL
⅓ cup	hazelnut flour (see Tips, left)	75 mL
¼ cup	tapioca starch	50 mL
1 tsp	xanthan gum	5 mL
½ cup	butter	125 mL
1 cup	white chocolate chips	250 mL
2	eggs	2
½ cup	granulated sugar	125 mL

TOPPING

¾ cup	apricot jam	175 mL
1 cup	white chocolate chips	250 mL
¼ cup	sliced hazelnuts	50 mL

1. *Base:* In a bowl or plastic bag, combine rice flour, hazelnut flour, tapioca starch and xanthan gum. Mix well and set aside.

2. In a small saucepan over low heat, melt butter and white chocolate chips, stirring constantly until melted. Set aside.

3. In a separate bowl, using an electric mixer, beat eggs and sugar until thick and creamy, about 5 minutes. Stir in melted chocolate mixture and dry ingredients. Mix well.

4. Spread half the batter in prepared pan with a moist rubber spatula. Set remaining batter aside. Bake base in preheated oven for 20 to 25 minutes or until lightly browned. Cool for 5 minutes.

5. *Topping:* Spread jam over base. Stir white chocolate chips into remaining batter. Drop by spoonfuls evenly over the jam. Spread out gently with moist rubber spatula. Sprinkle with hazelnuts. Bake for 30 to 40 minutes longer or until set. Cool completely, then cut into squares.

Nanaimo Bars

MAKES 3 DOZEN BARS

9-inch (2.5 L) square pan, lightly greased

Named for the city on Vancouver Island in British Columbia, Canada, these no-bake squares are family favorites in our households.

TIPS

A 1-oz (30 g) envelope of custard powder contains ¼ cup (50 mL).

∾

One individually wrapped square of baking chocolate equals 1 oz (30 g).

VARIATIONS

Substitute gluten-free white cake crumbs, almond flour or pecan flour for hazelnut flour. To make your own hazelnut flour, see Techniques Glossary, page 179.

∾

For a more traditional thick glaze, melt together 3 to 4 oz (90 to 120 g) semi-sweet chocolate and 1 tbsp (15 mL) butter. Substitute an equal amount of instant vanilla pudding mix for custard powder.

BASE

⅓ cup	butter, melted	75 mL
1	egg	1
1 tsp	vanilla extract	5 mL
⅓ cup	unsweetened cocoa powder	75 mL
2 tbsp	granulated sugar	25 mL
2 cups	hazelnut flour (see Variations, left)	500 mL
1 cup	unsweetened desiccated coconut	250 mL
½ cup	chopped walnuts	125 mL

FILLING

¼ cup	butter, softened	50 mL
3 tbsp	milk	45 mL
¼ cup	GF custard powder (optional) (see Tips, left)	50 mL
2 cups	GF sifted confectioner's (icing) sugar	500 mL

GLAZE

1 tsp	shortening	5 mL
1 to 2 oz	semi-sweet chocolate, cut into 6 pieces	30 to 60 g

1. **Base:** In a large bowl, blend together melted butter, egg and vanilla. Add cocoa, sugar, hazelnut flour, coconut and walnuts. Stir until combined. Spread evenly in prepared pan. Chill completely.

2. **Filling:** In a separate bowl, using an electric mixer, cream butter. Slowly add milk, custard powder, if using, and confectioner's sugar. Mix until combined. Spread over base and chill.

3. **Glaze:** In a small bowl, microwave shortening and chocolate on Medium for 1 to 2 minutes. Stir until completely melted. Drizzle in ribbons over chilled filling. Refrigerate before cutting into squares.

Equipment Glossary

Baking liners. Reusable sheets of nonstick coated fiberglass. Flexible and food-safe, they are used to eliminate the need to grease and flour. Wash, rinse well and dry before storing.

Bundt pan. A tube pan with fluted sides.

Cake tester. A thin, long, wooden or metal stick or wire attached to a handle that is used for baked products to test for doneness.

Cooling rack. Parallel and perpendicular thin bars of metal at right angles, with feet attached, used to hold hot baking off the surface to allow cooling air to circulate.

Cornbread pan. A cast iron corn-shaped pan with detailed construction that shows the kernels and ridges of seven ears of corn. The pan, which measures 11-by $5\frac{1}{2}$-inches (28 by 14 cm), can be used to make hot dog buns, cornbread buns or dinner rolls.

English muffin rings. Available in sets of four or eight $3\frac{3}{4}$ inch (8 cm) round, 1 inch (2.5 cm) high, these rings hold batter in place as it bakes.

Griddle. Flat metal surface on which food is cooked. Can be built into a stove or stand-alone.

Grill. Heavy rack set over a heat source used to cook food usually on a propane, natural gas or charcoal barbecue.

Hamburger bun baking pans. A baking pan that makes six 4-inch (10 cm) hamburger buns.

Hot dog bun baking pan. A baking pan that makes eight 6-by 2-inch (15 by 5 cm) buns to use for hot dogs or mini-submarine sandwiches.

Jelly roll pan. A rectangular baking pan, 15 by 10 by 1 inch (40 by 25 by 2.5 cm) used for baking thin cakes.

Loaf pan. Metal container used for baking loaves. Common pan sizes are 9 by 5 inches (2 L) and 8 by 4 inches (1.5 L). Danish loaf pans measure 12 by 4 by $2\frac{1}{2}$ inches (30 by 10 by 6 cm).

Parchment paper. Heat-resistant paper similar to waxed paper, usually coated with silicon on one side; used with or as an alternative to other methods (such as applying vegetable oil or spray) to prevent baked goods from sticking to the baking pan. Sometimes labeled "baking paper."

Pastry blender. Used to cut solid fat into flour, it consists of five metal blades or wires held together by a handle.

Pastry brush. Small brush with nylon or natural bristles used to apply glazes or egg washes to dough. Wash thoroughly after each use. To store, lay flat or hang on a hook through a hole in the handle.

Pizza wheel. A large, sharp-edged wheel (without serrations) anchored to a handle.

Ramekin. A small ceramic soufflé dish with a 4-oz (120 mL) capacity.

Rolling pin. A heavy, smooth cylinder of wood, marble, plastic or metal; used to roll out dough.

Scone pan. A $9\frac{5}{8}$-by 1-inch (22 by 2.5 cm) round metal baking pan portioned into eight sections; used to make scones by spooning in a drop batter.

Skewer. A long, thin stick (made of wood or metal) used in baking to test for doneness.

Spatula. A utensil with a handle and blade that can be long or short, narrow or wide, flexible or inflexible. It is used to spread, lift, turn, mix or smooth foods. Spatulas are made of metal, rubber or plastic.

Springform pan. A circular baking pan, available in a range of sizes, with a separable bottom and side. The side is removed by releasing a clamp, making the contents easy to remove.

Thermometers

• **Instant read thermometer.** Bakers use this metal-stemmed instrument to test the internal temperature of baked products such as cakes and breads. Stem must be inserted at least 2 inches (5 cm) into the food for an accurate reading. When quick bread is baked, it should register 200°F (100°C), yeast breads should register 190°F (95°C).

• **Meat thermometer.** Used to read internal temperature of meat. Temperatures range from 120°F to 200°F (60°C to 100°C). Before placing meat in the oven, insert the thermometer into the thickest part avoiding the bone and grizzle. If using an "instant read thermometer," remove meat from oven and test with thermometer.

• **Oven thermometer.** Used to measure temperatures from 200°F to 500°F (100°C to 275°C). It either stands on or hangs from an oven rack.

Tube pan. A deep round pan with a hollow tube in center, usually 10 inches (25 cm) in diameter, 16 cups (4 L) volume.

Zester. A tool used to cut very thin strips of outer peel from citrus fruits. It has a short, flat blade tipped with five small holes with sharp edges.

Ingredient Glossary

Almond. Crack open the shell of an almond and you will find an ivory-colored nut encased in a thin brown skin. With the skin removed (see Techniques Glossary, page 178), the almond is blanched. In this form, almonds are sold whole, sliced, slivered and ground. Two cups (500 mL) almonds weigh about 12 oz (375 g).

Almond flour (Almond meal). See Nut flour. (See Techniques Glossary, page 178 for directions to make.)

Amaranth. One of the oldest grains, amaranth flour is gluten-free. When stored in an airtight container, it has an indefinite shelf life.

Anise seeds. These tiny gray-green, egg-shaped seeds have a distinctive licorice flavor. Anise can also be purchased as a finely ground powder. For recipes that call for anise seeds, half the amount of anise powder can be substituted.

Arrowroot. It is referred to as a starch, a flour and as arrowroot starch flour. (Also see The Gluten-Free Bake Shop, page 9.)

Asiago cheese. A pungent grayish-white hard cheese from northern Italy. Cured for more than 6 months, its texture is ideal for grating.

Baking chips. Similar in consistency to chocolate chips, but with different flavors such as butterscotch, peanut butter, cinnamon and lemon.

Baking powder. Select gluten-free baking powder. A chemical leavener, containing an alkali (baking soda) and an acid (cream of tartar), which gives off carbon dioxide gas under certain conditions.

Baking soda (sodium bicarbonate). A chemical leavener that gives off carbon dioxide gas in the presence of moisture — particularly acids such as lemon juice, buttermilk and sour cream. It is also one of the components of baking powder.

Bean flour. See The Gluten-Free Bake Shop, page 9.

Bell peppers. The sweet-flavored members of the capsicum family (which include chilies and other hot peppers), these peppers have a hollow interior lined with white ribs and seeds attached at the stem end. They are most commonly green, red or yellow, but can also be white or purple.

Black bean flour. A high fiber gluten-free flour mainly used in Tex Mex dishes.

Blueberries. Wild low-bush berries are smaller than the cultivated variety, and more time-consuming to pick, but their flavor makes every minute of picking time worthwhile. Readily available year-round in the frozen fruit section of many grocery stores.

Brown rice flour. See The Gluten-Free Bake Shop, page 10.

Brown sugar. A refined sugar with a coating of molasses. It can be purchased coarse or fine and comes in three varieties: dark, golden and light.

Buckwheat. Also known as saracen corn. Not related, despite its name to wheat (which is a grain), buckwheat is the seed of a plant from the rhubarb family. Buckwheat flour is dark with a strong pungent flavor and is gluten-free. Buckwheat groats are the hulled seeds of the buckwheat plant. Soft white seeds with a mild flavor that when roasted or toasted the flavor intensifies. Roasted whole buckwheat, called kasha, has a strong nutty flavor and chewy texture.

Butter. A spread produced from dairy fat and milk solids, butter can be used interchangeably in quick bread recipes for shortening, oil or margarine.

Buttermilk. Named for the way in which it was originally produced — that is, from milk left in the churn after the solid butter was removed — buttermilk is now made with fresh, pasteurized milk that has been cultured (or soured) with the addition of a bacterial culture. The result is a slightly thickened dairy beverage with a salty, sour flavor similar to yogurt. Despite its name, buttermilk is low in fat.

Caraway seeds. Small, crescent-shaped seeds of the caraway plant. They have a nutty, peppery, licorice-like flavor.

Cardamom. This popular spice is a member of the ginger family. A long green or brown pod contains the strong, spicy, lemon-flavored seed. Although native to India, cardamom is used in Middle Eastern, Indian and Scandinavian cooking — in the latter case, particularly for seasonal baked goods.

Cassava. See Tapioca Starch in The Gluten-Free Bake Shop, page 10.

Cheddar cheese. Always select an aged or old, good-quality Cheddar for baking recipes. (The flavor of mild or medium Cheddar is not strong enough for baking.) Weight/volume equivalents are:
4 oz (120 g) = 1 cup (250 mL) grated;
2 oz (60 g) = ½ cup (125 mL) grated;
1½ oz (45 g) = ⅓ cup (75 mL) grated.

Coconut. The fruit of a tropical palm tree with a hard woody shell that is lined with a hard white flesh. Three forms available can be sweetened or not: flaked, shredded and the smallest desiccated (thoroughly dried).

Corn flour. A flour that can be milled from the entire kernel of corn. Corn flour and cornstarch are not interchangeable in recipes. Freeze corn flour to prevent molds developing.

Cornmeal. The dried ground kernels of white, yellow or blue corn. It has a gritty texture and is available in coarse, medium and fine grind. It is the coarser grind of corn flour and cornstarch. Check label of commercial products for addition of wheat. Maizemeal can be corn or wheat. Its starchy-sweet flavor is most commonly associated with cornbread — a regional specialty of the southern United States.

Cornstarch. See The Gluten-Free Bake Shop, page 9.

Corn syrup. A thick, sweet syrup made from cornstarch, sold as clear (light) or brown (dark or golden) varieties. The latter has caramel flavor and color added.

Cranberry. Grown in bogs on low vines, these sweet-tart berries are available fresh, frozen and dried. Fresh cranberries are available only in season — typically from mid-October until January, depending on your location — but can be frozen right in the bag. Substitute dried cranberries for sour cherries, raisins or currants.

Cream of tartar. It is used to give volume and stability to beaten egg whites. It is also an acidic component of baking powder. Tartaric acid is a fine white crystalline powder that forms naturally during the fermentation of grape juice on the inside of wine barrels.

Cross-contamination. The process by which one product comes in contact with another one that is to be avoided. For example, toasters, oven mitts, cutting boards and knives, when used for products containing gluten, still have gluten on them, which is passed on to the gluten-free product. You must either have separate tools or be sure that the gluten is washed off completely before being used by people with gluten sensitivity.

Currants. Similar in appearance to small, dark raisins, currants are made by drying a special seedless variety of grape. Not the same as a type of berry that goes by the same name.

Dates. The fruit of the date palm tree, dates are long and oval in shape, with a paper-thin skin that turns from green to dark brown when ripe. Eaten fresh or dried, dates have a very sweet, light-brown flesh around a long, narrow seed.

Eggs. Liquid egg products, such as Naturegg Simply Whites, Break Free and Omega Pro liquid eggs and Just Whites, are available in Canada and the U.S. Powdered egg whites such as Just Whites can be used by reconstituting with warm water or as a powder. A similar product is called meringue powder in Canada. Substitute ¼ cup (50 mL) liquid egg product for 1 large egg.

Egg replacer. A powder that is used in place of eggs, which acts as a leavening agent. Reconstitute according to package instructions.

Egg substitute. A liquid made from egg whites or reconstitute dried egg whites according to package instructions.

Eggplant. Ranging in color and shape from dark purple and pear-like to light mauve and cylindrical, eggplant has a light, spongy flesh that, while bland on its own, is remarkable for its ability to absorb other flavors in cooking.

Evaporated milk. A milk product with 60% of the water removed. It is sterilized and canned, which gives it a cooked taste and darker color.

Fava bean flour. See Bean Flour in The Gluten-Free Bake Shop, page 9.

Fennel seeds. Small, oval green-brown seeds with prominent ridges and a mild anise (licorice-like) flavor and aroma. Available whole or ground, they are used in Italian and Central European cookery, particularly in rye or pumpernickel breads.

Feta cheese. A crumbly, white Greek-style cheese, with a salty, tangy flavor. Store in the refrigerator, in its brine, and drain well before using. Traditionally made with sheep or goat's milk in Greece and usually cow's milk in Canada and the U.S.

Fig. A pear-shaped fruit with a thick, soft skin, available in green and purple. Eaten fresh or dried, the tan-colored sweet flesh contains many tiny edible seeds.

Filbert. See Hazelnut.

Flaxseed. Thin and oval shaped, dark brown in color, flaxseed add a crunchy texture to baked products. Research indicates that flaxseed can aid in lowering blood cholesterol levels. Ground flaxseed (also known as linseed) stales quickly, so purchase only the amount needed. Store in the refrigerator. It acts as a tenderizer for yeast breads. It can be used with or without eggs and adds omega-3 oil and fiber. Flaxseed should be cracked or ground to be digested.

Garbanzo bean flour. See Bean Flour in The Gluten-Free Bake Shop, page 9.

Garbanzo-fava flour. See Bean Flour in The Gluten-Free Bake Shop, page 9.

Garfava flour. See Bean Flour in The Gluten-Free Bake Shop, page 9.

Garlic. An edible bulb composed of several sections (cloves), each covered with a papery skin. An essential ingredient in many styles of cooking.

Ginger. A bumpy rhizome, ivory to greenish-yellow in color, with a tan skin. Fresh gingerroot has a peppery, slightly sweet flavor, similar to lemon and rosemary, and a pungent aroma. Ground ginger is made from the dried gingerroot. It is spicier and not as sweet or as fresh. Crystallized or candied ginger is made from pieces of fresh gingerroot that have been cooked in sugar syrup and coated with sugar.

Gluten. A natural protein in wheat flour that becomes elastic with the addition of moisture and kneading. Gluten traps gases produced by leaveners inside the dough and causes it to rise.

Glutinous rice flour. See Sweet rice flour. Also see The Gluten-Free Bake Shop, page 10.

Golden raisins. See Raisins.

Granulated sugar. A refined, crystalline white form of sugar that is also commonly referred to as "table sugar" or just "sugar."

Guar gum. A white flour-like substance made from an East Indian seed high in fiber, this vegetable substance contains no gluten. It may have a laxative effect for some people. It can be substituted for xanthan gum.

Half-and-half cream. The lightest of all creams, it is half milk, half cream with a butterfat content between 10 and 18%. It can't be whipped, but is used with coffee, or on cereal. To substitute, use equal parts cream and milk OR evaporated milk OR $7/8$ cup (210 mL) milk plus $1\frac{1}{2}$ tbsp (22 mL) butter or margarine.

Hazelnut. Also known as filberts, hazelnuts have a rich, sweet flavor that complements ingredients such as coffee and chocolate. Remove the bitter brown skin before using.

Hazelnut flour (Hazelnut meal). See Nut flour, page 180.

Herbs. See also individual herbs. Plants whose stems, leaves or flowers are used as a flavoring, either dried or fresh. To substitute fresh herbs for dried, a good rule of thumb is to use three times the amount of fresh as dried. Taste and adjust the amount to suit your preference.

Honey. Sweeter than sugar, honey is available in liquid, honeycomb and creamed varieties. Use liquid honey for baking.

Kasha. See Buckwheat.

Linseed. See Flaxseed.

Maple syrup. A very sweet, slightly thick brown liquid made by boiling the sap from North American maple trees. Use pure maple syrup in baking, not pancake syrup.

Margarine. A solid fat derived from one or more types of vegetable oil. Do not use low-fat margarines in baking, since they contain too much added water.

Mesclun. A mixture of small, young, tender salad greens such as spinach, frisée, arugula, oak leaf and radicchio. Also known as salad mix, spring mix or baby greens and sold pre-packaged or in bulk in the grocery produce section.

Millet. A small seed of a cereal grass or grain closely related to corn. With a nutty aroma and taste, it is an excellent source of fiber and moderate source of protein.

Molasses. A byproduct of refining sugar, molasses is a sweet, thick, dark-brown (almost black) liquid. It has a distinctive, slightly bitter flavor and is available in fancy and blackstrap varieties. Use the fancy variety for baking unless blackstrap is specified. Store in the refrigerator if used infrequently.

Nonfat dry milk. See Skim milk powder.

Nut flour (Nut meal). A flour made by finely grinding nuts such as Almond flour, Hazelnut flour or Pecan flour. To make, see Techniques Glossary, page 180.

Olives (Kalamata). A large, flavorful variety of Greek olive, typically dark purple in color and pointed at one end. They are usually sold packed in olive oil or vinegar.

Olive oil. Produced from pressing tree-ripened olives. Extra virgin oil is taken from the first cold pressing; it is the finest and fruitiest, pale straw to pale green in color, with the least amount of acid, usually less than 1%. Virgin oil is taken from a subsequent pressing; it contains 2% acid and is pale yellow. Light oil comes from the last pressing; it has a mild flavor, light color and up to 3% acid. It also has a higher smoke point. Product sold as "pure olive oil" has been cleaned and filtered; it is very mild-flavored and has up to 3% acid.

Parsley. A biennial herb with dark green, curly or flat leaves used fresh as a flavoring or garnish. It is also used dried in soups and other mixes. Substitute parsley for half the amount of a strong-flavored herb such as basil.

Pea flour. See The Gluten-Free Bake Shop, page 9.

Pecan. The nut of the hickory tree, pecans have a reddish, mahogany shell and beige flesh. They have a high-fat content and are a milder-flavored alternative to walnuts.

Pecan flour (Pecan meal). See Nut meal. For instructions how to make, see Techniques Glossary, page 180.

Pistachio nut. Inside a hard, tan-colored shell, this pale green nut has a waxy texture and mild flavor.

Poppy seeds. The tiny, round blue-gray seed of the poppy has a sweet, nutty flavor. Often used as a garnish or topping for a variety of breads.

Potato flour. See Potato starch.

Potato starch (Potato starch flour). See The Gluten-Free Bake Shop, page 10.

Pumpkin seeds. Hulled and roasted green pumpkin seeds have a nutty flavor that enhances many breads. In Mexico, where they are eaten as a snack and used as a thickener in cooking, they are also known as pepitas.

Quinoa. It is the most nutritious grain available, high in protein, calcium and iron content. The small seeds look like millet and are naturally coated with a bitter tasting saporin to protect it from birds and insects. Quinoa flour is gluten-free with a delicate, nutty taste. It makes a moister, higher-fat product. Quinoa flour can be substituted for rice flour in most recipes.

Rhubarb. A perennial plant with long, thin red- to pink-colored stalks, resembling celery and large green leaves. Only the tart-flavored stalks are used for cooking, since the leaves are poisonous. For 2 cups (500 mL) cooked rhubarb, you will need 3 cups (750 mL) chopped fresh, about 1 lb (500 g).

Raisins. Dark raisins are sun-dried Thompson seedless grapes. Golden raisins are treated with sulphur dioxide and dried artificially, yielding a moister, plumper product.

Rice flour. See The Gluten-Free Bake Shop, page 10.

Rice Bran. See The Gluten-Free Bake Shop, page 10.

Sesame seeds. Small, flat, oval-shaped seeds with a rich, nut-like flavor when roasted. Purchase the tan (hulled), not black (unhulled), variety for use in baking.

Shortening. A partially hydrogenated, solid, white flavorless fat made from vegetable sources.

Skim milk powder. The dehydrated form of fluid skim milk. Use ¼ cup (50 mL) skim milk powder for every 1 cup (250 mL) water.

Sorghum flour. Also known as Jowar. See The Gluten-Free Bake Shop, page 10.

Sour cream. A thick, smooth, tangy-flavored product made by adding bacterial cultures to pasteurized, homogenized cream containing varying amounts of butterfat. Check the label, some low-fat and fat-free brands may contain gluten.

Soy flour. See The Gluten-Free Bake Shop, page 10.

Starch. Starch is found in the cells of plants and insoluble in cold water. When cooked, the granules swell and thicken or gel.

Sugar substitute. For baking, the best choice is sucralose, which is made from processed sugar and remains stable at any temperature.

Sun-dried tomatoes. Available either dry or oil-packed, sun-dried tomatoes have a dark red color, soft chewy texture and strong tomato flavor. Use dry, not packed in oil, sun-dried tomatoes in recipes. Use scissors to snip.

Sunflower seeds. Use shelled, unsalted, unroasted sunflower seeds in bread recipes. If only roasted, salted seeds are available, rinse under hot water and dry well before using.

Sweet peppers. See Bell peppers.

Sweet potato. A tuber with orange flesh that stays moist when cooked. Not the same as a yam, although yams can substitute for sweet potatoes in recipes.

Sweet rice flour. See The Gluten-Free Bake Shop, page 10.

Tapioca starch. See The Gluten-Free Bake Shop, page 10.

Tarragon. An herb with narrow, pointed, dark green leaves and a distinctive anise-like flavor with undertones of sage. Use fresh or dried.

Vegetable oil. Common oils used are corn, sunflower, safflower, olive, canola, peanut and soy.

Walnuts. A sweet-fleshed nut with a large wrinkled shell.

Wild rice. In its natural state it's gluten-free but when found in boxed wild rice/white rice mixes, it's best avoided. To cook see Techniques Glossary, page 180.

Xanthan gum. A natural carbohydrate made from a microscopic organism called Xanthomonas campestris, this gum is produced from the fermentation of glucose. It is used to add volume and viscosity to baked goods. Used as an ingredient in gluten-free baking to give the dough strength, thus allowing it to rise and prevent it from being too dense in texture. It does not mix with water, so must be combined with dry ingredients. Purchase from bulk or health food stores.

Yeast. See The Gluten-Free Bake Shop, page 11.

Yogurt. Made by fermenting cows' milk using a bacteria culture. Plain yogurt is gluten-free, but not all flavored yogurt is.

Zest. Strips from the outer layer of rind of citrus fruit. Used for its intense flavor.

Techniques Glossary

Almonds. *To blanch:* Cover almonds with boiling water and allow to stand, covered, for 3 to 5 minutes. Drain. Grasp the almond at one end, pressing between your thumb and index finger and the nut will pop out of the skin. Nuts are more easily chopped or slivered while still warm from blanching. *To toast:* see Nuts, page 180.

Almond flour or **Almond meal.** *To make:* See Nut flour (Nut meal), page 180.

Baking pan. *To prepare or to grease:* Either spray the bottom and sides of the baking pan with a nonstick cooking spray or brush with a pastry brush or a crumpled up piece of waxed paper dipped in vegetable oil or shortening.

Bananas. *To mash and freeze:* Select overripe fruit, mash and package in 1 cup (250 mL) amounts in freezer containers. Freeze for up to 6 months. Defrost and warm to room temperature before using. About 2 to 3 medium bananas yield 1 cup (250 mL) mashed.

Barbecue by indirect method. To cook with the heat source coming from one or both sides of the food and not directly beneath it.

Beat. Stir vigorously to incorporate air using a spoon, whisk, hand-beater or electric mixer.

Blanch. Food is completely immersed in boiling water and then quickly in cold water to loosen and easily remove the skin.

Blend. Mix two or more ingredients together thoroughly, with a spoon or using the low speed of an electric mixer.

Bread crumbs. *To make:* For best results, the GF bread should be at least one day old. Using the pulsing operation of a food processor or blender, process until crumbs are of consistency desired. To store, package in airtight containers and freeze.

Cake crumbs. See Bread crumbs.

Caramelize onions. See Onions.

Chocolate. *To melt:* Chop each 1 oz (30 g) square into 4 to 6 pieces. Place in a heat-proof bowl or the top of a double-boiler over hot water to partially melt the chocolate. Remove from heat and continue stirring until completely melted.

Coconut. *To toast:* See Nuts.

Combine. Stir two or more ingredients together for a consistent mixture.

Cream. Technique of combining softened fat and sugar by beating to a soft, smooth creamy consistency while trying to incorporate as much air as possible.

Cream cheese. *To warm to room temperature:* For each 8-oz (250 g) package, cut into 1-inch (2.5 cm) cubes, arrange in a circle on a microwave-safe plate and microwave on High for 1 minute.

Cut in. Technique used for combining solid fat and flour until the fat is the size required (for example, like small peas or meal). Use either two knives or a pastry blender.

Dredge. A step in the breading process that coats a food with flour or bread crumbs before frying. This enables the batter to adhere to the food more easily.

Drizzle. Slowly spoon or pour a liquid (such as frosting or melted butter) in a very fine stream over the surface of food.

Dust. Coat by sprinkling GF confectioner's (icing) sugar, cocoa powder or GF flour lightly over food or a utensil.

Eggs. *To warm to room temperature:* Place eggs in the shell from the refrigerator in a bowl of hot water and allow to stand for 5 minutes.
To warm egg whites to room temperature: Separate eggs while cold. Place in a bowl of hot water and allow to stand for 5 minutes.

Envelope fold. *To make:* Place food off center on double thickness of heavy-duty foil. Bring long end up and over food loosely causing all edges to meet. Seal edges with two to three $\frac{1}{2}$-inch (1 cm) folds. Be sure to pinch the folds tightly so any steam created is sealed in the package. Care must be taken not to put a hole in the package during cooking.

Flaxseed. *To grind:* Place whole seeds in a coffee grinder or blender. Grind only the amount required. If necessary, store extra ground flaxseed in the refrigerator.
To crack: Pulse in a coffee grinder, blender or food processor just long enough to break the seed coat but not grind completely.

Fold. Gently combine light whipped ingredients with heavier without losing the incorporated air. Using a rubber spatula, gently fold in a circular motion. Move down one side of the bowl and across the bottom, fold up and over to the opposite side and down again turning bowl slightly after each fold.

Garlic. *To roast:* Cut off top of head to expose clove tips. Drizzle with $\frac{1}{4}$ tsp (1 mL) olive oil and microwave on High for 70 seconds or until fork-tender. Or bake in a pie plate or baking dish at 375°F (190°C) for 15 to 20 minutes.
To peel: Use the flat side of a sharp knife to flatten the clove of garlic. Then skin can be easily removed.

Glaze. Apply a thin, shiny coating to the outside of a baked, sweet or savory food to enhance the appearance and flavor

Grease pan. See Baking pan.

Griddle. *To test for correct temperature:* Sprinkle a few drops of water on the surface. If the water bounces and dances across the pan, it is ready to use.

Hazelnuts. *To remove skins:* Place hazelnuts in a 350°F (180°C) oven for 15 to 20 minutes. Immediately place in a clean, dry kitchen towel. With your hands, rub the nuts against the towel. Skins will be left in the towel. Be careful: hazelnuts will be very hot.

Hazelnut flour or **Hazelnut meal.** *To make:* See Nut flour (Nut meal), page 180.

Herbs. *To clean fresh leaves:* Rinse under cold running water and spin-dry in a lettuce spinner. If necessary, dry between layers of paper towels. Place a dry paper towel along with the clean herbs in a plastic bag in the refrigerator for short-term storage. Freeze or dry for longer storage.
To dry: Tie fresh-picked herbs together in small bunches and hang upside down in a well-ventilated location with low humidity out of sunlight until the leaves are brittle and fully dry. If they turn brown (rather than stay green), the air is too hot. Once fully dried, strip leaves off the stems for storage. Store whole dried herbs in an airtight container in a cool dark place for 1 year and dried crushed herbs for 6 months. Dried herbs are stored in the dark to prevent the color from fading. Check herbs and discard any that have faded, lost flavor or smell old and musty.
To dry using a microwave: Place $\frac{1}{2}$ to 1 cup (125 to 250 mL) of herbs between layers of paper towels. Microwave on High for 3 minutes, checking often to be sure they are not scorched. Microwave for extra 15-second periods until leaves are brittle and can be pulled from stems easily.
To freeze: Lay whole herbs in a single layer on a flat surface in the freezer for 2 to 4 hours, leave whole and pack in plastic bags. Crumble the leaves directly into the dish. Leaves of herbs are also easier to chop when frozen. Use frozen leaves only for flavoring and not garnishing as they lose their crispness when thawed. Some herbs such as chives have a very weak flavor when dried and do not freeze well but they do grow well inside on a windowsill.
To measure: Remove small leaves from stem by holding the top and running fingers down the stem in the opposite

direction of growth. Larger leaves should be snipped off the stem using scissors. Pack leaves tightly into correct measure.
To snip: After measuring, transfer to a small glass and cut using the tips of sharp kitchen shears/scissors to prevent bruising the tender leaves.
To store: Fresh picked herbs can be stored for up to 1 week with stems standing in water. (Keep leaves out of water.)

Mix. Combine two or more ingredients uniformly by stirring or with an electric mixer on a low speed.

Nut flour (Nut meal). *To make:* Toast nuts (see Nuts, below), cool to room temperature and grind in a food processor or blender to desired consistency.
For ground nuts: Bake at 350°F (180°C) for 6 to 8 minutes and grind finer.

Nuts. *To toast:* Spread nuts in a single layer on a baking sheet and bake at 350°F (180°C) for about 6 to 8 minutes, shaking the pan frequently, until fragrant and lightly browned. (Or microwave uncovered on High for 1 to 2 minutes, stirring every 30 seconds.) Nuts will darken upon cooling.

Olives. *To pit:* Place olives under the flat side of a large knife; push down on knife until pit pops out.

Onions. *To caramelize:* In a nonstick frying pan, heat 1 tbsp (15 mL) oil over medium heat. Add 2 cups (500 mL) sliced or chopped onions; cook slowly until soft and caramel-colored. If necessary, add 1 tbsp (15 mL) water or white wine to prevent sticking while cooking.

Peaches. *To blanch:* See Blanch.

Pecan flour or **Pecan meal.** *To make:* See Nut flour (Nut meal), above.

Pumpkin seeds. *To Toast:* See Sunflower seeds.

Raisins. *To plump:* Measure spirit (usually brandy) into liquid measuring cup and add raisins; microwave on High for 1 minute and allow to cool.

Sauté. Cook quickly in a small amount of fat at high temperature.

Sesame seeds. *To toast:* See Sunflower seeds.

Sunflower seeds. *To toast:* Spread seeds in a single layer on a baking sheet and bake at 350°F (180°C) for 10 minutes, shaking pan frequently, until lightly browned. (Or microwave uncovered on High for 1 to 2 minutes, stirring every 30 seconds.) Seeds will darken upon cooling.

Whip. Beat ingredients vigorously to increase volume and incorporate air, typically using a whisk or electric mixer.
Whip eggs to soft peaks: Egg whites beaten to a foam that comes up as the beaters are lifted and fold over at the tips.
Whip eggs to stiff peaks: Egg whites beaten past soft peaks until the peaks remain upright when the beaters are lifted.

Wild rice. *To cook:* Rinse $\frac{1}{3}$ cup (75 mL) wild rice under cold running water. Add along with 2 cups (500 mL) water to a large saucepan. Bring to a boil and cook uncovered at a gentle boil for about 35 minutes. Reduce heat, cover and cook for 10 minutes or until rice is soft but not mushy. Makes 1 cup (250 mL). Store in refrigerator for up to 1 week.

Zest. *To zest:* Use a zester, fine side of a box grater or small sharp knife to peel off thin strips of the colored part of the skin of citrus fruits. Be sure not to remove the bitter white pith below.

American Celiac Groups

Celiac Sprue Association
402-558-0600
Fax: 402-558-1347
Website: www.csaceliacs.org

Celiac Disease Foundation (CDF)
13251 Ventura Boulevard, Suite 1
Studio City, California 91604-1838
818-990-2354
Fax: 818-990-2379
Website: www.celiac.org

The Gluten Intolerance Group of North America (GIG)
15110-10th Avenue SW, Suite A
Seattle, Washington 98166-1820
206-246-6652
Fax: 206-246-6531
Website: www.gluten.net

American Celiac Society/Dietary Support Coalition
59 Crystal Avenue
West Orange, New Jersey 07052
Email: AmerCeliacSoc@netscape.net

CSA/USA, Inc.
PO Box 31700
Omaha, Nebraska 68131-0700

Raising Our Gluten-Free Kids (R.O.C.K.)
Website: www.celiacKids.com

Celiac Disease and Gluten-Free Diet Support Page
Website: www.celiac.com

Celiac Support Groups in the United States
Website: www.enabling.org/ia/celiac/groups/groupsus.html

Canadian Celiac Association Chapters

NATIONAL OFFICE
5170 Dixie Road, Suite 204
Mississauga, ON L4W 1E3
905-507-6208
1-800-363-7296
Fax: 905-507-4673
Email: celiac@look.ca
Website: www.celiac.ca

ALBERTA
Calgary Chapter
4112-4th Street N.W.
Calgary, AB T4K 1A2
403-237-0304
Fax: 403-269-9626

Edmonton Chapter
Room 5R17
11111 Jasper Avenue
Edmonton, AB T5K 0L4
Tel/Fax: 780-482-8967
Website: www.celiac.edmonton.ab.ca

BRITISH COLUMBIA
Kamloops Chapter
116 River Road
Kamloops, BC V2C 1L9
250-374-6185
Email: egordon@mail.ocis.net

Kelowna Chapter
2468 Thatcher Road
Kelowna, BC V2C 4P9
250-763-1935
Email: celiac_kelowna@hotmail.com

Vancouver Chapter
1212 Broadway West, Suite 306
Vancouver, BC V6G 3V1
604-736-2229
Fax: 604-730-1015
Email: ccavancouver@canada.com
Website: www.vcn.bc.ca/celiac

Victoria Chapter
PO Box 5765, Station B
Victoria, BC V5R 4G8
250-472-041
Email: victoriaceliac@canada.com

MANITOBA
Winnipeg Chapter
PO Box 2543
Winnipeg, MB R3C 4B3
204-772-6979
Website: www.celiac.mb.ca

NEW BRUNSWICK
Fredericton Chapter
527 Beaverbrook Court, Ste. 226
Fredericton, NB E3B 1X6
506-450-4357

Moncton Chapter
PO Box 1576
Moncton, NB E1C 9X4

Saint John Chapter
454 Elmore Crescent
Saint John, NB E2M 3C1
506-672-4454

NEWFOUNDLAND
St. John's Chapter
262 Freshwater Road
St. John's NF A1B 1B8
709-753-6766

NOVA SCOTIA
Halifax Chapter
114 Woodlawn Road
Halifax, NS B3K 5M7
902-435-9019
Website: www3.ns.sympatico.ca/celiac.halifax

ONTARIO
Hamilton Chapter
PO Box 65580
Dundas Postal Outlet
Dundas, ON L9H 6Y6
905-572-6775

Kingston Chapter
551 Rankin Crescent
Kingston, ON K7M 7K6
613-389-6776

Kitchener/Waterloo Chapter
153 Frederic Street, Suite 118
Kitchener, ON N2H 2M3

London Chapter
PO Box 198
Dorchester, ON N0L 1G0
Email: celiaclondon@golden.net

Ottawa Chapter
Box 39035, Billings PO
Ottawa, ON K1H 1A1
613-786-1335
Website: www.celiac.ottawa.on.ca

Peterborough Chapter
195 London Street
Peterborough, ON K9H 2Y8
705-740-9784

Quinte Chapter
PO Box 20104
Belleville, ON K8N 5V1

St. Catherines Chapter
Grantham PO Box 20193
St. Catharines, ON L2M 7W7

Sudbury Chapter
PO Box 2794, Stn. A
Sudbury, ON P3A 5J3

Thunder Bay & District Chapters
PO Box 1102, Station F
Thunder Bay, ON P7C 4X9
807-475-3800

Toronto Chapter
PO Box 27592, Yorkdale PO
Toronto, ON M6A 3B4
416-781-9140

PRINCE EDWARD ISLAND
Charlottetown Chapter
PO Box 2291
Charlottetown, PEI C1A 8C1

QUEBEC
Quebec Chapter
4887 Boul. De Maissonneuvre Ouest
Westmount, QC H3Z 1M7

SASKATCHEWAN
Regina Chapter
PO Box 1773
Regina, SK S4P 3C6

Saskatoon Chapter
PO Box 8935
Saskatoon, SK S7K 6S7

National Library of Canada Cataloguing in Publication

Washburn, Donna
125 best gluten-free recipes / Donna Washburn and Heather Butt.

ISBN 0-7788-0065-2

1. Gluten-free diet—Recipes. 2. Celiac disease—Diet therapy—Recipes. I. Butt,
Heather II. Title. III. Title: One hundred twenty-five best gluten-free recipes.

RC862.C44W38 2003 641.5'631   C2002-905890-2

Index